DEB

When you wake
on how to live and who to be,
remember that by being you,
I am me.

Thank you for being you.

This is true for you and your
family especially. ACN were years
that planted in me a spirit of
confidence I hadn't experienced in
years. Wouldn't be possible without
you, Deb.

I hope a story or idea from these
pages touch your heart and you share
that feeling with someone you love.

xoxo

MAN, YOU KNOW I GOT YOU

Advanced Praise

"Jonathan is like a brother. And this conversation about men's mental health is near and dear to my heart. It's so important for men to know that they are not alone. I know Jonathan's work with Project Circle Up and this book will make a positive impact in the way men talk, think, and feel about their mental health and masculinity. This is a must read."
—*Kurtis Gabriel,* Canadian Professional Ice Hockey Player for the Toronto Maple Leafs

"Jonathan Andrews' story is powerful, heartwarming, and inspiring. He is truly a man of purpose who understands how his story can help people across the world. He embodies the title, "Man, You Know I got you" in every way."
—*Aimé Mukendi Jr. AKA "Sir Aimézing,"* International Speaker & Best Selling Author of, "Everyone Needs a Hero: Why Can't it be you?"

"'Man, you know I got you' is a candid, emotional real take on men's mental health. Exploring narratives and hardships men often experience alone while providing a road map to wellness and healthy living we desperately need right now."
—*Mike Shoreman,* Mental Health Advocate, Award Winning Speaker, Author, Athlete

"This book should be required reading for ALL men. Jonathan's powerful and vulnerable storytelling lifted a weight off my spirit and reminded me that I'm never alone in my struggles. This book will pave the way for the future of men's mental health discussions. Reading it was like speaking to a brother who truly loves and cares about you."
—*SAM DEMMA,* Award-Winning Youth Speaker and Entrepreneur

A great piece of work that provides solidarity around coping with mental health. Men tend to be more of a closed book when discussing these topics but 'Man, you know I got you' is a book you must open to feel the presence of an author who understands the world of mental health on an extremely relatable level."
—*Cole Rowden,* CEO Etho Ventures

"As an Arab man, I find this text to not only encompass the hard pill our generation of men have had to swallow for decades, but a manual to discovering the strength in opening up to the real issues inside. Jonathan's art in expression makes him unique and relatable to millions of men across all walks of life, especially for those needing the assurance in knowing their feelings and struggles are valid. I pray that men get to share this text with one another knowing where real strength lies: together."

—*Ally Salama*, Forbes 30 Under 30, CEO EMPWR, Empathy Always Wins Podcast, Ex-Pro Athlete, and The Middle East's Mental Health Ambassador

MAN, YOU KNOW I GOT YOU

WHY THE FUTURE OF MEN'S MENTAL HEALTH AND MASCULINITY ARE NOT "MAN UP" BUT CIRCLE UP

JONATHAN ANDREWS

Hardcover: 987-1-7773736-4-1
Ebook: 978-1-7773736-5-8

First paperback edition November 2021.

Edited by Tabitha Rose & Flor Ana Mireles
Cover art and images by Alejandro Baigorri
Layout by Arash Jahani
Interior Design by Brady Moller

Life to Paper Publishing
Toronto, Canada | Miami, U.S.

www.lifetopaper.com

"Cherish your visions. Cherish your ideals.

Cherish the music that stirs in your heart, the beauty that forms in your mind, the loveliness that drapes your purest thoughts.

For out of them will grow all delightful conditions, all heavenly environment, of these, if you but remain true to them, your world will at last be built."

James Allen, As a Man Thinketh

This book is dedicated to Noah Jackson Andrews

You taught me more about grief, love, and my mental health than any words can describe.

Did I leave the world better than I found it?

Man can anchor his entire existence in this fundamental question.

The earth?

Your children?

The surf?

Your decision.

The ripples of daily action touch shores beyond comprehension.

A simple deed

righteous and kind

its depths unknown

its lasting effects were blind.

When you wake tomorrow and reflect on how to live and who to be

remember that by being you, I am me.

23/03/2020 - 05/04/2020

RIP

FOREWORD:

As Founder & Executive Director of Jack.org, Canada's only charity training and empowering young leaders to revolutionize mental health, it has been a joy and an inspiration to watch Jonathan Andrews take his personal experiences, heartbreak, and challenges and turn them into incredible action, change, and leadership. Particularly with respect to helping young men learn about and engage in the topic of mental health.

First, some background. The story behind Jack.org, where I had the good fortune to meet Jonathan, starts with tragedy. My wife Sandra Hanington and I, with the support of our family and closest friends, founded what would become Jack.org in 2010, after we found out that our eldest son Jack had died by suicide during his first year of university. We were shocked and absolutely devastated, especially as we had no idea that Jack was even struggling. We thought we were a very happy, healthy, and fortunate family. Once the clouds started to part, we immediately set out to find out how this could have happened. The fact that mental health is the biggest health challenge for our youth, and that suicide is the leading health-related cause of death of our youth, became quickly apparent. To pay honour to Jack, and to make sure some good came from our loss, we started our journey to help transform the youth mental health landscape in Canada. Our ambition was to ensure that no family would ever have to go through what we did. Fast forward to today, our staff of over 60 works with thousands of incredible young leaders, like Jonathan, to break down barriers to positive mental health and advocate for change in their communities, and across the country. All of our approximately 3,000 youth volunteers are incredible in their own right, and Jonathan stands out as a leader among these inspiring young advocates. Especially when it comes to bringing this conversation to young males, who, like Jack, have been conditioned to "be quiet ", "suck it up ", and tend to not be open to either sharing their struggles or learning how to support themselves or their peers.

One of our core principles at Jack.org is "Youth Front and Centre ", which has enabled me to learn from so many incredible young leaders like Jonathan. Using his lived experience, empathy, and significant skills, Jonathan has paved the way for so many young men who don't have strong examples of the type of masculinity that this book outlines - masculinity that is based in vulnerability, community, and knowing that you're not alone. He saw the crisis facing men and their mental health, and wanted to make a lasting difference.

I'll never forget sharing the stage with Jonathan in 2017. We had never met, were three decades apart in age, and had different life experiences. But hearing him speak, I immediately knew that we were bonded through a common goal: to make the change that we wanted to see in the world of youth mental health. I am so grateful to have been able to witness Jonathan continue to fight, advocate, educate, and lead every day since.

Through his work with Jack.org, and now Project Circle Up, Jonathan is showing more men every day that it is okay to take off your mask and "feel ". No longer should young men be taught to "man up ", but rather they should "circle up ", by coming together, being vulnerable, and learning how to support themselves and their peers. I was so honored to be able to attend a Project Circle Up session and see for myself the transformation that is starting with these young men. They are actively living the principles that Jonathan lays out in his book - being there for one another, embracing their pain and their joy, and giving each other permission to be their truest selves.

It is crucial for young men to start to understand that they are not alone, that it is okay to seek help, and that they do not have to conform to the ideals of manhood they have been conditioned to exhibit. Jonathan's work, and the book you are about to read, lays the groundwork for a new era in men's mental health. I'm so grateful for Jonathan, for this heartfelt and insightful contribution to our shared passion of youth mental health, and for all of the young men who are going to carry the torch and "circle up "for one another after reading Man, You Know I Got You.

Eric Windeler
Founder & Executive Director
Jack.org

Table of Contents

INTRODUCTION

"You must not write what you want or would like to write. It must be what you *have* to write. Write that without which you could not live."

Christopher Hitchens

You Are Not Alone

If you've ever felt lost and directionless, you're in good company. If you've ever felt depressed, welcome to the club. And if you've ever wondered if this life is worth it or thought about suicide, you're not alone. When I was a boy, the world was my oyster. I was athletic, driven and even liked by girls. My possibilities seemed endless. Until they weren't. In high school, I suffered a devastating downward spiral. Medically diagnosed with clinical depression, I was on the verge of drowning. This is a glimpse into my story.

Dean was a close family friend. I played hockey with his son. He helped my dad build our deck. Hell, he even made my grandpa's dentures.Then, one day, my teacher sat me down in the library beside two of my best friends to break the news. Dean was found in his garage, hanging from a rope. It was the first time that a man in my life would kill himself. At the time, most of my friends and family seemed to grieve and move on, but I didn't. I felt small.

Problems that used to feel like ripples in the water—deadlines, peer pressure, girls—began to feel like tidal waves. At the time, I was thinking to myself, "How could this happen? I just saw you laughing. I just saw your smile. You looked and sounded fine, and, now, you're dead. "It was like, all of a sudden, the sun stopped shining for me. And then, I was just sad and the sadness was so consuming that I couldn't get away from it.

I started taking a knife to my arm, harming myself just to feel *something*. I felt so alone that I started picturing myself in the garage, taking Dean's place, dangling. When I was on the verge of drowning, my dad reached out to me and taught me the lesson that became the seed of the Circle Up movement. He showed me that I was not alone. I remember it like it was yesterday. That defining day started, as so many had at that point in my life, with my alarm going off at 7 a.m. and me unplugging it. My dad, like he had every day for months, came into my room desperate to get me out of bed and into class.

Our struggle lasted for over an hour. Back and forth and back and forth. Finally, he said, "I have fucking had it, "and stormed out of the room. Convinced I had won this round, I rolled over to go back to sleep. Then, he burst back into the room; this time with a big bucket of water and poured it all over me. "Holy shit! "That got me up. Then, he looked me in the eye and said something that later became the basis for everything we fight for and believe in at Circle Up.

My father said, "I cannot imagine what you're going through, but I promise to sit right here for as long as you need. You are not alone. You will never be alone."

I am alive today because that man fought for me. That day, and all the months that followed. That first struggle with my mental health opened my eyes to a bigger picture. Exasperated and amplified by the global health pandemic of 2020, men have never been lonelier, felt more lost or full of doubt. Today, a man is killing himself every minute of every day and it's clear we can no longer ignore that the state of our men's mental health has become a global crisis. In my eyes, it's Dean and his family's memory, as well as the memory of every man we've lost, that gives Circle Up the strength to fight back.

We fight back by supporting Jack.org and the movement for youth mental health education. We fight back by leading weekly men's circle's—where men don't have to just "man up "or struggle alone, because we give a fuck about each other. And we fight back, in the same way you can, by sharing my dad's gift. The gift of a committed listener. The gift of a safe space. The gift of knowing that someone gives a damn. That you're not alone.

Today, all I want is to be the man my dad was for me, for the men in my life. Because of him, I know that it only takes one person who cares enough to change the world.

The Purpose Of This Book

The purpose of this book is to be part of helping men change the way they think, feel, and act on their mental health. Instead of "man up, "we can Circle Up by cultivating, and investing in, empowered masculine relationships. These men become brothers, as they have for me, in the pursuit of discovering and dissolving the barriers holding you back from well-being, finding and living your purpose, and from happiness. Collectively we take action towards the men we've always wanted to be, knowing that becoming this man is our greatest gift to the world. There's going to be ideas and concepts in these pages that you disagree with. And that's okay. Just don't throw the baby out with the bathwater.

Jim Rohn made an excellent point in his famous lectures when he would say, "Don't be a follower, be a student. Take what I say and process it, think about it, ponder it. If it makes you think, it's valuable. Then, when you take action, make sure the action is the product of your own conclusions. "If you agree with what we cover together, you'll know why. If you don't, consider those ideas to be a conduit for introspection. The questions that will make this book valuable to your life are:

1. **What does what I'm reading reveal about who I am as a man?**
2. **What can I learn about myself through this concept?**
3. **What opportunities are there for me to think, be, or act differently that would help me on my path to being the man I've always wanted to be?**

If you come away from this book learning something about yourself, it will prove to be an extremely valuable investment in your personal development. Further, let it be a tool reminding you, and the men in your life, that whether you're lost or directionless, depressed, or wondering if this life is worth it and thinking of suicide, that you're not alone. The more I learn about masculinity, the more clearly I see that most men, including myself, have been conditioned to believe that alone means strong. Self-made means resourceful, and needing, asking for, and considering help, makes you weak and less of a man. This couldn't be further from my truth.

This positioning of masculinity, as we'll explore more deeply in chapter one, is destroying our men, and thereby, our families and communities. I believe, as a result of my own struggles with mental health, through countless interactions with young people in schools across Canada, and through my participation and leadership of men's circles over the last three years, that reprogramming the "man up" belief system to a Circle Up mentality, has the potential to unlock more positive change in our men's mental health than any other current opportunity. ☯[1]

In so many ways, we're the luckiest generations to ever live. In others, we face unique and tremendous challenges. Even with our advancements in Science, Technology, and Manufacturing, global discrimination, abuse, and inequality, on both the systemic and individual levels, seem to persist. And it was our aim in this book, and in our programs at Circle Up, to tackle these challenges at the level of the root cause, rather than via their symptoms. With this

1 ☯ **Philosophy Footnote:** *"If you want to go fast, go alone. If you want to go far, go together."* - **African Proverb**

book, therefore, I hope to be part of discovering and dissolving the barriers of disconnection, segregation, and fear that have men, and humans collectively, choosing ego and intelorence before commitment and love.

According to the World Health Organization (WHO), a man dies by suicide every minute. That's over 500,000 men every year. You can likely bring to mind a handful of men in communities you've been part of who've died by suicide. I personally know dozens of men who've killed themselves since Dean's death. My closest friends in the world have lost their fathers, and some of my greatest mentors and role models have lost their sons and brothers. Hoping things will get better, or that the Government will take care of our wellbeing, is no longer an approppropriate strategy. While I'm hopeful they have good intentions, they've proven incapable.

Eckhart Tolle, Spiritual Teacher and Author of the worldwide bestseller *The Power of Now*, wrote, "If you find your here and now intolerable and it makes you unhappy, you have three options: remove yourself from the situation, change it, or accept it totally."

Knowing the suffering I've felt personally, and the pain I've witnessed in my best friends and their families, I see no alternative than to be part of the change we want to see for men's mental health and masculinity. Because, if not now, when? If not you and I, who?

This book, as well as the founding of Circle Up as a virtual men's circle, it's ongoing program delivery and evolution over time, represent our stand for a different life. A resolve that enough good men have been lost. That we will no longer be silent while our brothers suffer alone. And that we will change the way men think, feel, and act on men's mental health and masculinity.

We know that a future exists where men can come together and give a fuck about each other. We know this because we're seeing the evolution before our eyes. This book, and our effort at Circle Up, is only possible as a result of standing on top of the shoulders of giants: the men who've come before us and have dedicated their lives to digging the well of our better future. If you're called to, I invite you to use this book as continued fuel to be part of this movement to stand for our men's mental health, and as a result, the wellbeing of their families and our communities.

What This Book Is About And What Will You Learn

While science and research played a huge role in the writing and development of this book, it is not intended to be an academic research paper. It's an operating manual. You'll find wisdom and practical advice that you can apply to your life as we discuss how to dissolve the current inherited beliefs we tend to hold around men's mental health and masculinity and give you a roadmap to:

1. **Why men struggle with their mental health**
2. **How men are able to hide their struggle from even their closest friends and family**
3. **What to do about the men's mental health crisis we now face**

Virtually, all of these ideas, philosophies, and lessons have been around for thousands of years. So if there's any credit I can assume in this book, it's simply for interpreting them through my own life experience and synthesizing them in a way that's highly actionable.

More broadly, this book is about masculine relationships and about how to differentiate between where, when, and with whom it's appropriate to have these difficult conversations with, because they're not always appropriate. Most importantly, this book, and the Circle Up movement, are about how to intentionally create the conditions and relationships where you can discuss anything you're struggling with in your life. Relationships where even your darkest demons can be on the table. Where you know without a shadow of a doubt the space is trusted and confidential. And with the men who remind you that you're never alone. I can say with conviction that, when you find and cultivate this environment, your life will never be the same.

These ideas have proven effective for me in my pursuit of becoming self-sufficient and purpose driven, but this book is no Bible. You will find concepts that can be applied immediately to generate massive positive results in your life. You will equally find ideas that create internal conflict and that you disagree with. Pay attention to both. My intention moving forward is for you to take the risk of thinking for yourself. ☯[2]

WHAT THIS BOOK IS NOT

1. This book is not a replacement for professional mental health support

This book, and by extension, our programs at Circle Up, are not substitutes for professional care with your mental health. Chapter 4 outlines a spectrum so that you can decide what actions are appropriate based on the state of your mental health now. Additionally, we do not explore in great detail in this book the impact mental illness has on a man's mental health. And so, in the cases of a severe struggle or crisis with mental health, as well as a severe mental illness, I encourage you to seek professional care.

None of our leaders are medical practitioners and none of the ideas outlined in this book should replace the guidance of a trained mental health professional. Instead, you will find that a community like Circle Up is the perfect place to come, if you're willing, in order to find the metaphorical mirror you've been missing. Similar to the Master Mind outlined in texts like Napoleon Hill's *Think and Grow Rich*, our community can act as a mirror reflecting back to you what we see and hear. Inside a masculine environment that includes trust and confidentiality, you may finally see the blind spots that have been there all along. You may finally see your own bullshit.

---

2 ☯ **Philosophy Footnote:** *"Take the risk of thinking for yourself... Don't seek refuge in the false security of consensus."* - **Christopher Hitchens**

2. This book is not a clinical analysis of neuroscience, psychotherapy, or mental illness

While we will help provide a new context for looking at mental health, we're not teaching the academics of these fields of study. In this book, you will not find an in-depth review of the anatomy, biochemistry, or molecular biology of the brain, the nervous system, or how and why mental illness manifests.

We focus on, and deal primarily with, the forgotten and lost aspects of what it means to be a man. If you've ever asked yourself, "How do I be a man in a world of toxic masculinity? "or "Where were the lessons on integrity in school? "or "What is my life purpose? "or are confused on the principles and values that make us men, this book is for you. ☯[3]

3. This book is not a magic pill

If you let it, the Circle Up community, and this book, can assist you in doing the necessary introspection to change your life. There is no guarantee that by reading this book or by participating in a Men's Circle that your life will change for the better, and here's why: firstly, in order for you to see what the primary excuses and reasons you use to let yourself off the hook in your life, you'll need to be honest with yourself.

As men, we wear masks, (defined in detail in chapter two) and, as a result of trying to protect our ego, we find ourselves with an urgent desire to be right, to look good or avoid looking bad, and to maintain our current status quo (even though we may say we want to change or the conditions of our lives are painful). Until you can choose truth over comfort, there is little this book, or Circle Up, can do to help.

Further, just because you reveal your blindspots to yourself does not mean that you will do anything differently. So if you're looking for the ideas in this book, or the men on your men's team to change your life, you will be disappointed. We can provide you with new tools to apply to your life and be the mirror that helps reveal you to yourself,

---

3 ☯ **Philosophy Footnote:** *"It is important to disentangle our societal notions of 'toxic masculinity' from our notions of 'masculinity.' This way, we can connect with our nature and masculinity in a healthy way that serves us." - Iain Gabriel.*

but doing the work to become the man you've always wanted to be, is, and has always been, in your hands.

Transformation Is Possible

I often think about the boy who hadn't been to class in months, who couldn't get himself to shower, who smoked weed all day and cut himself, and my heart swells with pride. I'm so grateful for that kid. For finding strength, for breaking the toxic habits that had him spiralling downwards, but most of all, for accepting and asking for help. That expression of humility allowed him to take off his mask of masculinity long enough to be cared for by those who loved him. ☯[4]

In the proceeding 10 years since my clinical depression diagnosis, self-harming, and thoughts of suicide, my life has transformed. While I'm in no way perfect at following the principles and philosophies outlined in this book—and often fall into the traps of old ways of thinking, feeling, and acting, such as telling the men in my life I am fine when I'm lying—I've made enough progress to confidently share the ideas that transformed my life and the lives of countless men who come in search of solutions in our programs at Circle Up. ☯[5]

For a moment, consider the transformation you're seeking. What has changed? What relationships have you let go of? What thoughts will you no longer embrace? What habits have you developed and what actions do you now take? Who have you become as a man? Certainly everyone's progress will look different, but as you decide whether or not to invest your time and energy into this book, let me paint a picture of possibility and give you an example of my personal transformation. This is what is waiting for you and the men in your life on the other side of directionlessness and doubt.

---

4 ☯ **Philosophy Footnote:** *"The broken heart is what allows the light to come in."* **- Rumi**

5 ☯ **Philosophy Footnote:** *"The thinker without paradox is like the lover without emotion."* **- Kierkegaard**

After accepting help with my mental health in high school, developing a desire to change my life, and taking action towards a better future, I graduated College and went on to land my dream job and make (and save) hundreds of thousands of dollars before I was twenty-three years old. While working, I began serving as a volunteer with Canada's leading youth mental health charity, Jack.org. During that time, I had the honour of representing their brand by giving over a hundred speeches at High Schools, Universities and businesses all across Canada with the mission of helping those communities change the way they talk, think and feel about mental health.

My new ways of thinking and acting in the world have helped me gain my confidence back and become self-sufficient. I've dated women whom I never thought I could have had a chance with, and these women continue to change my life and make me a better man. I've road tripped across Canada, traveled all over the world, and, as of this writing, have stopped focusing on making a living and paying rent and instead have begun focusing on designing a life I love surrounded by the people I love. My current plans have me three months into a global Vagabond with my best friend Iain and any of our amigos who take us up on the offer.

Now, if any of this sounds like I'm bragging, that's not my intention. I share my own story of transformation to prove to you that it's possible. And that getting out of your comfort zone, whether that's starting a conversation about mental health with one of your friends, beginning the discipline of doing ten push-ups every day, or any number of infinite steps you could take in the direction of your better mental health, is worth it. James Allen, in his book, *As a Man Thinketh* wrote, "The will to do stems from the knowledge that you can do."

My small example is just one of hundreds of men I know personally who made a decision to change their lives for the better and fucking did it. Some of their stories include losing fifty pounds, starting the businesses of their dreams, and saving their marriages from the brink of destruction. I want you to know, and have faith that, whatever the transformation you're seeking, is possible. You're not alone on this journey.

A Note On Philosophy Footnotes: Meet Iain

Iain, a man you will hear about plenty in this book, is my best friend. He is also responsible for all of the philosophy footnotes you will observe throughout the book. When I was getting ready to edit, my brother Jeremy gave me sound advice that I should find someone who knows my voice. No one knows me better than Iain. So I asked him to help edit this text and he agreed.

As we sat together over many days in a writer's paradise, a secluded shack located on a nature reserve during Guatemala's rainy season, Iain's brain simply wouldn't stop coming up with quotes, concepts, and additional thoughts that related to what I had written. Therefore, we have included them for your introspection in the footnotes. In my eyes, and in those of the people who know Iain intimately, he is a genius. He is the unique intersection of when being unapologetically yourself, meets brilliant mind, meets the desire to be self-expressed and make a useful contribution to the world. I joke in earnest that he is my personal philosopher and I have happily shared the gift he has had in my life with you here. Enjoy!

CIRCLE UP

Beyond the money, and beyond the travel, what I'm most proud of throughout my journey has been the brothers I've gained along the way. These men (you know who you are), the ones who have my back, who create opportunity for me, and most importantly, who call me out on my bullshit for not living the principles outlined in this book, are the reason I continue this work.

On numerous occasions since Dean took his own life, I've experienced trauma and loss, and instead of retreating into myself as I did as a boy, I call my men. I remember my dad's lesson that we're never alone and I allow the men in my life to show up and care for me. It's because of these men, I've learnt to trust. Instead of bottling up my emotions, I've learned to feel them, process them, and let them go.

I am eternally grateful for these brothers who continue to give a fuck about me. It's because of these men that I am a better man for myself, my family and everyone else I love and care about. If at any point throughout the book you feel compelled to reach out and participate in Circle Up or to simply learn more, message us:

Instagram: **@projectcircleup or @jonathanfandrews**
Email: **jonathanandrewscircleup@gmail.com**
Website: **circleup.ca**

In many ways this entire book is simply an introduction. It's an introduction to me, to Circle Up, and to the broader challenges we as men face in respect to our mental health and masculinity.

In his advice to young writers, Christopher Hitchens said, "You must not write what you want or would like to write. It must be what you have to write. Write that which without you could not live."

This book exists because I could no longer live without writing it.

My whole heart is in this text and I hope the stories, philosophy, and ideas serve as the foot in the door to your thriving mental health and a new way of thinking, feeling, and acting on your masculinity. The real work begins when you close this book, step outside, and start a conversation about what you want to do and who you want to become.

Jim Rohn once shared, "Your life, my life, each of our lives, is going to serve as either a warning or an example. A warning of the consequences of neglect; self pity; and lack of direction and ambition. Or as an example of talent, put to use; discipline, self imposed; or of objectives clearly perceived and intensely pursued."

While this book and this community can be part of your supporting cast, only you have the power to change your life.

So with that, I invite you to take the first step. Reach out to us and read on. While the first step is always the most difficult, I'm confident that, when you take it, life will be so full of colour and love and abundance that you'll never look back.

Don't "man up, "Circle Up!

Playa del Carmen, México - January 2021

PART ONE

MAKING THE UNCONSCIOUS, CONSCIOUS

CHAPTER ONE:

WHY MEN STRUGGLE WITH MENTAL HEALTH

"Until you make the unconscious conscious, it will direct your life and you will call it fate."
Carl Jung

Our Uniting Force

Early in my personal development journey, I heard a fable about a journalist who was tasked with interviewing two virtually opposite men: one a criminal, the other a wealthy businessman. The first, abused drugs, was in and out of jail his whole life, and was broke living on welfare. The second man lived a beautiful life. He was wealthy, he cherished his family, and was respected by his entire community. The only similarity was they were twin brothers. So when the newspaper owner heard their story, he immediately sent a journalist to understand how two brothers, who grew up in the same environment, with virtually identical genetics, could live such completely opposite lives.

It turned out that their father was also a criminal. He was the root cause of incredible pain throughout their home. He abused drugs, his wife, and his two sons. The first brother, who was serving time for armed robbery, blamed his father for setting a terrible example. When asked, "How did your life turn out this way? "He answered, "With a father like mine, how could it turn out any other way? "The second brother, who was being recognized internationally for his successful businesses, agreed that his father set a terrible example for his family.

But when asked, "How did your life turn out this way? "He answered, "With a father like mine, how could it turn out any other way? "

In this example, two sons with the same environment, virtually identical genetics, and the same abusive father, went on to live completely different lives. The first, repeated the blueprint laid out by their dad. The second, became the molder and shaper, instead of the slave, of his circumstances. One, limited by the memories of the past. The other, defined by a vision of the future.

This chapter is about the first brother. It's about the belief systems, unconscious programming, and barriers we face as men, that hold us back from becoming the men we've always wanted to be. Once we understand why men struggle, we can talk about how they get away with it so easily, and then, what we can do about it.

Although there are dozens of reasons why men struggle with their mental health and why suicide has become a global crisis, let's explore three of them together:

1. **Many of the assumptions that we hold to be true about our mental health and masculinity aren't workable**
2. **We experience trauma and don't heal from it**
3. **We live most of our lives in our heads**

Our Beliefs About Men's Mental Health And Masculinity

Reflecting on my years as a teenager struggling with depression, three major analogies exposed to me why I had gone from a kid with all the promise in the world to experiencing suffering and wanting to end my life. The first was described by the late great business philosopher Jim Rohn: "Think of your personal philosophy as the sail on a sailboat. It's not the blowing of the wind that determines your destination, it's the set of your sail. "

"The same wind blows on us all, "Jim would say. "The wind of disaster. The wind of opportunity. The wind of change. The social wind, the political wind, the economic wind. The difference in where you arrive, therefore, is not in the blowing of the wind but in the set of the sail."

Jim showed me, like with the story of the two twin brothers, the hardship you experience (the wind) matters much less in how your life turns out than what you do about it (the set of your sail).

Another way to look at this concept of personal philosophy was introduced to me by a man who's changed hundreds of thousands of men's lives for the better through his seminars, Justin Sterling.

What do you see when you look at this picture?

At first glance, it just looks like a finger. But consider how many different interpretations there are for one image. In the context of your body, it's a finger. But in the context of numbers, it's one. And in the context of direction, it's up. Therefore, Justin revealed to me, the actions and decisions we make as men will all be determined depending on how we look at and perceive the world around us. We live our lives depending on our context.

Why does this matter?

The reason your context, or the set of your sail is so important, is that, no matter where you are or who you're with, what you do is determined by the set of your sail or how you look at your life.

This is also the reason why men's mental health has become a global crisis. The way we look at ourselves, our relationships with other men, as well as the way we look at the world, doesn't fucking work. Let me put it to you the same way it was put to me, bluntly. If you or a man in your life are not currently getting the results you want—either because you're broke, you're in a toxic relationship, or your mental and physical health is deteriorating—it is not because of what's happened to you, the wind, or your circumstances. The reason is because of the set of your sail. It's the way we look at what happens or our own personal philosophy, as Jim pointed out, that makes the difference in how our life turns out.

Unless you change how you are, you'll always have what you've got. Therefore, the bad news is that in order for your life to change, you need to change. What are the specific thoughts, feelings, and actions that led you to your current circumstances? I can't know for sure. That is why Circle Up exists as a personal development opportunity for men. It's a circle of confidentiality for men to come and uncover what it is about their personality that has created their depression, financial challenges, or relationships issues.

The good news, however, is that while it's not easy to rewire your beliefs, you can do it. ☯[6] I did it. And men all over the world are doing it every day. The result in my life change was dramatic. I was depressed, anxious, and on the verge of a mental health crisis. Now, I have money in the bank, purpose and meaning in my life, and I'm designing a life on my own terms. Nothing externally changed for me to arrive here. My transformation was not a change in the wind, but a change in how I set my sail.

Those changes in your sail need to start with your thinking. As Einstein pointed out, "We cannot solve our problems with the same thinking we used when we created them. "The same thoughts will always lead you to the same actions, which will always lead you to the same results. This brings us to the final analogy that facilitated my life change. All of my grandparents used to be enthusiastic gardeners and so when Jim Rohn used a farmer to describe the law of sowing and reaping, I paid attention.

Jim Rohn would say, "Whatever you reap is what you've sown."

When the farmer walks onto the field in the spring and plants kale, he's not going to harvest pumpkins in the fall. If he sows seeds of kale, he's going to reap harvests of kale. Jim showed me that our minds work the same way. Think of the seeds you plant as your thoughts, and the fruits you harvest as your results.

---

6 ☯ **Philosophy Footnote:** *"The will to do stems from the knowledge that one can do."*
- James Allen.

If you're planting seeds in the soil of your mind that money is scarce, that you're not good enough, and that struggling with your mental health makes you weak and less of a man, the fruits you harvest in the fall are going to be damaged, rotten, and toxic. However, if you plant thoughts of gratitude, love for yourself and the people in your life, and that you're committed to honouring how you feel with men that you trust, you will reap results of abundance of money, love and friendship, and thriving mental health.

What do these analogies and ways of thinking reveal about the fruit that is the state of men's mental health? Well, today, men who struggle don't seek help, but instead cope with drugs, sex, and pornography. 75% of suicides in Canada are committed by men. And, every minute, a man dies by suicide. Therefore, the clear answer to our crisis is that we're reaping what we've sown.

In 1903, James Allen wrote in *As a Man Thinketh*, "You are today where your thoughts have brought you; you will be tomorrow where your thoughts take you."

So, why do men struggle? We struggle because of our thoughts. Mental health literally refers to the health of our minds, the health of our thinking. And we struggle because our current cultural beliefs about men's mental health and masculinity have limitations. A resource I wish existed earlier and now offer to you is James Clear's *Atomic Habits*. My biggest personal take away was that, over time, our beliefs become essentially invisible to us. Our responses to these beliefs are so deeply encoded that we live most of our lives on autopilot.

So, it's for this reason that, in order for us to begin the process of behaviour change and the process of changing our thinking, we must start with awareness. We need to ask ourselves, what sail have I set? What context do I hold about mental health? What seeds am I planting in my mind? In his book, James Clear showed that to effectively build a new life, we need to first pay attention to the beliefs that run our day. This can be more challenging than it sounds because once a belief is firmly rooted in your life, it is mostly unconscious and automatic. The standout concept from the book that applies to why men struggle with their mental health is that, "If a belief remains mindless, you can't expect to improve it."

Then, I got goosebumps as he read a quote by Carl Jung that I feel summarizes the aim of this entire chapter in one profound sentence, "Until you make the unconscious conscious, it will direct your life and you will call it fate."

I had to hit rock bottom in my teens before I started paying attention to my belief systems. That experience with depression forced me to ask myself the same questions I'm now asking you:

- **What do I believe about myself and the world that created my current results?**
- **What does masculinity mean to me?**
- **Where did these beliefs come from?**

After years of introspection, hearing the stories of thousands of students in schools all across Canada, as well as years of being a participant and a leader of men's circles, these are the three most common beliefs about men's mental health and masculinity I've come across:

1. **Only crazy people have issues with their mental health**
2. **Struggling with my mental health makes me weak and less of a man**
3. **I need to "man up" when I'm stressed or struggling with my mental health**

These beliefs are based on stories and anecdotes from men's lives as well as my own lived experience with mental health struggle. Where we will focus this discussion is that these beliefs are not working. In the short term, these beliefs actually serve men because we get to avoid pain and move towards pleasure. Think, developing a drinking habit to numb the pain of losing a loved one. In the short-term, you feel good and get to avoid the pain and grief, but over the long-term, this type of thinking and these types of coping strategies have proven disastrous.

After Dean took his own life, I didn't talk about my anxiety because I believed that my depression made me weak. I wanted to stop hurting and start feeling good and so I started smoking more and more weed. And because I bought into the "man up "philosophy, I hid my pain from my friends and family.

Being questioned about my anxiety made me feel worse and so I slowly distanced myself from anyone that cared. In only a few weeks, I was skipping class and getting high every day. In a few months I stopped hanging out with my friends. And, eventually, the only things I could get myself to do was play video games, smoke weed, and sleep. At twenty-one years old, however, after years of distance from my depression, I started talking about my mental health for the first time because I realized that my experience wasn't unique.

This cycle is extremely common when we observe men and grieving, men and substance abuse, and men and mental health. As men, we experience stress or trauma and don't have outlets designed for us to process and move through them. We believe our struggle makes us weak and so we don't want anyone to see it. Instead of talking about it, we put on a mask and often cope with drugs and short-term pleasures.

All of a sudden, we find ourselves addicted, struggling, and don't know where to turn or who to talk to. Instead of facing the hole we've dug ourselves in, we pretend we're okay and begin the process all over again. The key here is not to judge ourselves or other men for demonstrating this behaviour. The key is to change the way we think about and feel, as well as act, on men's mental health so that we can have empathy, create spaces to have mental health conversations, and, ultimately, give a fuck about each other. As James Clear clearly outlined in *Atomic Habits*, the first step to change isn't judgement. It's awareness.

We Experience Trauma And Don't Heal From It

Another major reason men struggle with their mental health is that we experience stress and trauma in our lives, but we never heal from it. In order to explain this concept, I want you to briefly imagine yourself as a warrior. In Steven Pressfield's bestselling book, *The Warrior Ethos*, he said that wars change, but warriors don't. The more I consider this, the more useful this warrior analogy becomes on my own mental health journey. He explained that just because we're no longer storming beaches, doesn't mean we're not on battlefields. Even though wars look different today, what makes us warriors hasn't changed.

In the past, when a warrior would experience trauma, it would look like breaking a bone, losing an arm, or having an arrow pierce through their body. Today, because our battlefields look different, we still take arrows, they just happen to take shape mostly as mental, emotional, and psychological wounds. As a student, your battlefield may look like needing a certain grade to get you into the school of your dreams. As a working professional or business owner, your battlefield may look like making enough money to help your family get ahead. Or maybe, you found yourself with a substance abuse problem and your battlefield is getting sober.

In all three examples, the warrior will face stress in the form of obstacles, resistance, and defeat. Moreover, while you're fighting the good fight, the modern warrior will also experience trauma in unexpected ways, like your house burning down, going bankrupt, or the sudden death of a loved one. This adversity isn't a scrape of the knee or a broken wrist. These traumas can feel like an arrow piercing through your shoulder and sometimes even like a massive spear driving right through your chest.

If that seems like an exaggeration or false parallel, consider the tough loss of a loved one and how quickly you would have them back in exchange for an arrow in the arm.

As tragic and unfair as it all seems at the moment, this is the reality of the warrior. This is life. In the same way hiding your pain from the world by wearing a mask (a tool warriors use for protection) isn't the problem, taking arrows on the battlefield of your life isn't exclusively the reason why men struggle with their mental health.

As warriors, arrows go hand in hand with battle. The reason we struggle so deeply is that we get wounded, but never really heal. The opportunity for men isn't in learning how to avoid pain and tragedy, it is an inevitability. It's in the reconditioning of our relationship to the scraps, gashes, and the deep wounds of arrows. Jim Rohn joked about how it's only the men who we sit down in a corner, put a blanket over their heads, and give them three warm meals a day that will be able to avoid injury completely.

This overcaution is what he describes as one of the greatest diseases of attitude. "It's all risky! "he joked, "The minute you were born, it got risky. "He said, "If you think trying is risky, wait till they hand you the bill for not trying. Do you want to know how risky life is? You don't make it out alive. "

By nature the warrior inside of you wants a challenge. He wants an adventure. He wants to know that he'll be tested on the battlefield. Otherwise, what was all of the training and years of hard work and preparation for?

It's easy to think that, because of the negative emotions we've associated with hardship in the past, that, moving forward, we'd want only victories and positive experiences. I thought that way too, until I connected the warrior allegory to an example in one of my favourite books, *Busting Loose From The Money Game* by Robert Scheinfield. Being a warrior and never getting injured would be like:

"Scheduling the Superbowl between the Denver Broncos and the Seattle Seahawks, getting all of the players, coaches, referees, supporting staff, and fans at the stadium, having millions watching on television worldwide, then having the referee snap his fingers and say 'Ok, the Denver Broncos just won 37-10. You can all go home now.' The players don't want to go home. The coaches, referees, and support staff don't want to go home. The fans don't want to go home. Everyone wants all four quarters of the game to be played no matter what ups and downs might be experienced, how difficult the playing might get, or what the final outcome is. The players want to play because they love the game."

Even though we may say we don't want rejection and challenge and difficulty, the warrior spirit inside of us wants a fight. Despite the high chances of injury or even death, the warrior in you loves the battlefield. And so the problem lies not in the arrows, but in our inherited context around men's mental health.

The warrior, who knows the arrows go hand and hand with battle, doesn't shy away from them, but instead leans in and trains harder. He chooses the men he goes to battle with carefully. In the end, if he does get injured, which he will, he takes his wounds back to his men and they heal together. The ultimate confidence of a man is to know that, when faced with hardship, he will be okay.

Another important intersection between the warrior analogy and men's mental health is that the warrior knows it's in his best interest to have the men around him prepared, strong and healthy. Imagine running into battle where the man next to you couldn't raise his shield? You'd probably want to stand beside another man, wouldn't you? This context, coupled with the insight that every man will face injuries and trauma in his life, allows us to come together as men and be there for each other. In this way, rather than hide our arrows from the men around us, we can allow them to help us face our pain and heal, knowing that what's best for us, is best for them, and vice versa.

My best friend, Iain Gabriel, is, and will likely always be, my greatest personal test for how true I'm living this philosophy. He's so creative, charismatic, and cool that I often find myself jealous, resentful, and insecure around him. The beliefs that shape those behaviours are unconscious and don't serve me. We've been taught that resources are scarce and so we need to compete with other men.

The warrior analogy quickly allows me to reframe my insecurity to gratitude. Being around someone so outgoing as Iain, is like knowing that every time I step on the battlefield, I'm fighting side by side with Achilles or Leonidas of Sparta. Who else would you rather go to battle with than men who're strong, powerful, and take decisive action? When I focus on gratitude for having such an amazing man in my life, I stop trying to limit his success and instead begin investing in it. So much so that we joke in earnest that he is my personal philosopher. And further, he was instrumental in the editing, as well as is responsible for the powerful philosophy footnotes you see throughout this book.

The warrior context, if you're called to embrace it, shows you that ensuring the thriving health, wealth, and wellbeing of the men around you is actually the best thing you can do for your own mental wellbeing. You, and every man in your life, will face stress and even trauma. The opportunity of our generation is to transform our beliefs about these traumas from a story that creates division for fear that we will be perceived as weak and less of a man, to one that creates unity through the understanding that, as warriors, we're stronger together.

Losing a loved one and feeling like a massive spear just pierced through your heart is part of life and unavoidable. As Iain reminds me, "Pain is inevitable, suffering is a choice. "We have a choice moving forward to end the suffering. We can choose to face the trauma in our lives bravely, and, instead of wearing a mask and numbing ourselves with drugs, we can come together with our men and heal.

We Live Most Of Our Lives In Our Head

The final reason we will explore as to why men struggle with mental health is because fear has them living in their heads rather than in reality. You can think of the place men go when they stop taking action because they're consumed by anxiety, fear, and doubt as the basement.

My parents did everything they could to help me with my depression when I was a teenager. I was taking antidepressants, I was seeing counsellors at school and the hospital, and they showered me with love and support. Still, my anxiety and depression persisted for years. Why is that? Well, as we've discussed, my context about my mental health didn't work so instead of talking about it, I tried to hide my suffering and addiction. Further, Dean's death was a massive arrow that I never learned to heal or pull. I was slowly bleeding out. And lastly, as a result of these compounding factors, I was in the basement.

Think of your mental health like a house. From the top floor, or from thriving mental health, you have the best view. You have clarity in your vision, you often feel connected to your purpose, have meaning, and are taking action. The middle floor, or stress, is where we spend the majority of our time. We're going to work or school, we're managing our lives, and we're getting by. The basement, as you may have guessed, is where men go when they experience struggle and crisis.

Visually, the basement is a dark, cold, lonely place. Like a mouldy, unfinished and unfurnished cellar. The floors and the walls are made of concrete, the windows are boarded up, and there's no room for light, inspiration, or hope. It's the place warriors go when they've lost their will to kill. If you've ever experienced the basement, you know that sometimes it can feel like there's a ball and chain shackled to your leg.

The basement is where short-term coping strategies like drugs, sex, and over-indulgences are at their peak. The only reason we seem to be able to get off the couch is to grab another drink or take another hit. This place is also the point of maximum perceived separation and disconnection from the rest of the world.

When we're in the basement, rather than seeing that our struggle and our arrows connect us to the world, we allow our beliefs about men's mental health and masculinity to divide us, and this shouldn't come as a surprise. Our entire lives, we've been told that, if we're in the basement, it's a sign of weakness, and, to be a real man, you should hide your arrows from the world and just "man up." ☯[7]

I never understood the concept that vulnerability is strength until I realized how hard it is for a man in the basement to be honest about his situation. If you want a new way to look at manning up, consider it the strength to reach out for help. In 2018, I met a mentor whose personal philosophy revealed to me why so many men today are experiencing depression. Justin taught, "Doubt kills the warrior "and then added, so there was no room for misinterpretation, "Doubt kills the warrior. Because fear faced may cause injury, but the warrior lives to fight another day. It's doubt that men must beware."

I saved this for last because in respect to the basement and mental health struggle, I've yet to find a more simple and profound truth. When you're in the basement, you spend the majority of your life in your head. Doubt is so sinister because not only does it prevent men from taking action, but that inaction begins a cycle of more doubt followed by more inaction followed by more doubt, and, before you finish reading this sentence, men all over the world have talked themselves out of their dreams.

To explain this another way, Alan Watts pointed me to an analogy connecting this concept to the disturbing resonance created when a microphone gets too close to a speaker. I'm sure you can remember a time when you were in an audience and the sound system let out an intense and piercing screech. The closer the mic gets to the

---

7 ☯ **Philosophy Footnote:** *"In Art of Loving, Erich Fromm attributes all feelings of anxiety to a feeling or sense of separateness. From being apart from everyone else instead of being a part of everyone else. This feeling or sense of separateness is 'the illusion.'"* **- Iain Gabriel**

speakers the louder the resonance. The same thing happens to us when our predominant thoughts are of overwhelm, victimization, and hopelessness.

When we don't have the appropriate space designed for us to verbalize our negative thought patterns, they become further warped just like the microphone and speaker and begin to echo stronger and louder. In our men's circle, we call this echoing voice of doubt "monkeys." Seth Godin, author of dozens of best selling books, calls these monkeys the "lizard brain "and demonstrates that it's at the source of our debilitating self doubt.

It's hardwired into our genetics. And while this lizard brain is useful on a battlefield where a 6'7 dude with an axe is sprinting at you and about to murder your village, it's not helpful when you're about to ask a woman for her number or call a prospect at work. Men end up in the basement because they listen to that voice of resistance.

When you think of how great it would be to ask that cute girl for her phone number, but hear the echoing voice that she'd never be interested, that's the monkeys. When you consider how much it would help your family to ask for a raise at work, but the voice in your head says your boss will probably say no, that's the resistance. Or when you get the idea of starting a new workout program, but you convince yourself to start next monday, that's doubt and fear. Day after day, month after month, and year after year, men listen to that doubt and it's killing their warrior.

Slowly, like death by a thousand paper cuts, men descend deeper into the basement and sink heavier into their couches. Eventually, they can't stand up again. My best friend, Iain, reminds me that, "The problem most men face is not experiencing worry and anxiety. The problem is that we worry about worrying and get anxious about our anxiety. "This is exactly what I mean by men who live most of their lives in their head. The irony is that the same voice that lands most men in the basement is the same voice you can use as your greatest gift.

This voice, of course being the analytical mind, makes a great servant and a terrible master. Ultimately, men struggle with their mental health, not because they get wounded from their actions, but because they allow their doubt to take them off the battlefield. Remember that it's doubt, not action, that kills the warrior. Fear faced may cause injury, but the warrior gets to live and fight another day.

The butterflies you feel in your stomach reveal to you your edge. The tightness in your chest is a sign of your next opportunity for expansion. And taking action in the face of that fear is the metaphorical equivalent of taking a step up the stairs, out of the cold hopeless basement, and back into the light of day where you remember once again the beauty of a single breath and the magic of this moment.

CIRCLE UP

Up to this point, we've demonstrated that the reason men struggle is because they feel their mental health challenges make them weak and less of a man. ☯[8] That they need to put on a mask and hide their pain and arrows from the world. And because of the doubt that lands them on the couch and in their heads instead of on the battlefield taking action. When I meditate on how I went from depressed, addicted, and suicidal, to three years later thriving with my mental health and living the life of my dreams, I remember listening to the same two-hour Jim Rohn audio program a dozen times where he would say, "You cannot change the destination of your life overnight, but you can change the direction. "

The first step to any direction change is awareness, and we've done that here. Now that we know some of the "whys "of why men struggle with their mental health, we can take a look at the how. How do so many men struggle and get away with it? If we know that every minute a man dies my suicide, how come we haven't been able to

---

8 ☯ **Philosophy Footnote:** *"We need to address the faulty logic directly. If we accept the premise that a man having mental health issues makes him weak and less than a man, then almost every man in history is weak and less than a man. Part of realizing that you are not alone is realizing that you are not alone in your aloneness."* **- Iain Gabriel**

effectively intervene and do anything about it up to this point? Once we know the why and the how, we can talk about what to do about it.

As Carl Jung said, we've now made the unconscious conscious. The rest of this book is about taking fate into your own hands.

Circle Up!

Toronto, Canada - June 2020

Chapter Summary

Mental health struggles are like the fruit the farmer harvests in the fall. The fruit is a symptom. An outcome. The fruit, just like our struggle, is not the root. It is not the seed. So when we look at the fruit that is the state of our men's mental health: 75% of suicides are men, every minute a man dies by suicide, suicide is the #1 health related cause of death between 15-24, we must ask ourselves, what is the root? Why is there so much struggle? The answer to which is found in the quality of our thinking. The root of our men's mental health crisis stems from our beliefs and our perceptions about ourselves, masculinity and the world around us. You are not alone.

Resource Summary

Instead of looking through hundreds of links and book recommendations at the end of this book, I've provided you with a resource summary at the end of each chapter. This way you can stay close to the resources that are relevant to the concepts we discussed in the confines of a single theme, as well as take action on ideas, quotes, or thinkers you resonated most with in the moment. Pay attention to what speaks to your heart. If you say to yourself, "I should check that out, "take action immediately.

If you do not, the law of diminishing intent will squash that idea just as quickly as it arose. All you need from this book is one idea. A single idea could be enough to plant the seed of your future wealth, health, and happiness.

1. "Learn This Skill Or Live A Mediocre Life" - YouTube - Jim Rohn
2. Men's Weekend - Sterling-institute.com - Justin Sterling
3. The Ultimate Jim Rohn Library - Audible.com - Jim Rohn
4. As a Man Thinketh - James Allen
5. Atomic Habits - James Clear
6. The Warrior Ethos - Stevenen Pressfield
7. Busting Loose From The Money Game - Robert Scheinfield
8. Out of your mind - Audible.com - Alan Watts
9. Linchpin - Seth Godin
10. @iaingabriel - Instagram - Iain Gabriel

SELF-REFLECTION OPPORTUNITY

My recommendation is to create a note on your phone in order to capture the ideas worth filing, talking about, and implementing, all in one place. While the ideas are fresh, fill in the self-reflection opportunity below. Then, move all of the notes to your phone. This will serve to summarize what you have learned, as well as ensure the resources, quotes, and ideas you personally resonated with most, are available at your fingertips.

Key points to remember (fill in here):

What is one idea from this chapter that will help me "set a better sail" in my own personal philosophy?

CHAPTER TWO:
HOW MEN GET AWAY WITH MENTAL HEALTH STRUGGLE

"She had blue skin,
And so did he.
He kept it hid
And so did she.
They searched for blue
Their whole life through,
Then passed right by-
And never knew."

Shel Silverstein

WISHING WELL

The first time I felt like I fully understood how men get away with their mental health struggles was during my road trip across Canada in the Summer of 2020. Iain, my roommate and best friend, was and still is a huge Juice WRLD fan. At the time, he had been hyping the release of the upcoming posthumous album, *Legends Never Die*, since Juice's death in December of the prior year. Almost as if through divine intervention, the album was released just hours before we hit the road for our five-day drive from Toronto to British Columbia.

Midway through listening to the album, my ears perked up as the first lyrics of the hit song *Wishing Well* came out of the speakers. I had just started writing this book, and, as I listened, many of the themes I was hoping to communicate were present in the song. Juice WRLD sings about his deep desire to be free from his demons, his constant cycle of drugs and depression, and reveals a truth that virtually all men battle.

He sings:

> This is the part where I tell you I'm fine, but I'm lyin'
> I just don't want you to worry
> This is the part where I take all my feelings and hide 'em
> 'Cause I don't want nobody to hurt me

While listening to the expression of his pain and having nothing to do for hours but drive and think, I meditated on how many times I'd done the same thing on my mental health journey. Just like Juice WRLD, I realized that I too wore that same mask.

When I struggled with depression, I didn't want anyone to worry so I pretended everything was okay. That was my mask. When my dad confronted me that I was smoking weed every day, I acted as if it wasn't a problem. I hid the fact that I felt out of control, and that, even though I had tried several times to quit, I couldn't stop myself. My mask, again. Over and over, I wore the mask that communicated to everyone around me that I was okay, when my truth was I felt like I was drowning.

As Juice WRLD's tragic example has shown, we are really good at hiding our struggle. And for good reason. The masks we wear as men are evolutionary and instinctual. What started as one of our most important tools for success and achievement has now become one of the main reasons why our men struggle so desperately and get away with it. The purpose of this chapter is to highlight what masks are, why we wear them, and, most importantly, to reveal the main reason why they've become such a source of suffering for men globally.

WHAT ARE MASKS?

The concept of masks, borrowed from The Men's Weekend—a weekend seminar I attended in 2018—derives from the warrior allegory we explored in chapter one. Men on the battlefield would wear armor to give them strength and courage to fight, as well as protect them from an enemy sword or arrow. You can see that for the warrior, therefore, his armor was not only a matter of helping him become successful, but a matter of life and death.

Today, while our wars have changed, our warrior spirit has not. This analogy of wearing armor has transcended its use in war and become essential to modern man's success on the financial, relational, and emotional battlefields of his life. You and I wear masks in order to bring our best selves in business meetings, on the dance floor at the club, and at home with our families.

When I talk about masks I get two typical responses. The first is, "Of course. I wouldn't talk the same way on a date as I would with my mom. "And the second is a variation of, "I totally disagree. I value being genuine and authentic and try to never wear a mask."

Originally, I agreed with group two and felt that it was important for me to be consistent in every interaction. But that agreement was only intellectual. I soon changed my mind when I was challenged to spend a day becoming aware of my interactions. I quickly realized that every relationship dynamic is context dependent. Imagine you spoke to your boss the same way you spoke to your wife. Or that you hangout with your kids acting and being the same way you do when you are out at the bar drinking with your buddies. Different contexts bring out different parts of who you are.

I've even noticed that the tone of my voice changes subconsciously when I order a drink or food at a cafe or restaurant. Without even thinking about it, I put on my polite "Jonathan is ordering food now " mask. This doesn't mean that I'm a different person or that my value systems have changed; wearing masks often just means that you will naturally, and likely unconsciously, adjust how you interact with the world based on the context of the situation.

More often than not, when I share this concept, men don't disagree with the value of masks or that they wear one, they just don't like the word. If that is you, remember that the mask is just a symbol and a tool for communication. Many men prefer to think of masks simply being a tone, attitude, or way of being. Masks are not about being fake or inauthentic. Masks are a tool warriors use in order to gather strength, courage, and ensure they're able to protect their brothers going to battle with them, as well as their family and communities back at home counting on them to be successful.

It's also useful to understand other sources of origins of masks before they were muddied by the baggage that words and symbols can carry with them. In one of my favourite Alan Watts lectures on Audible *Out Of Your Mind,* he pointed out:

"Do you know that the word 'person' means 'mask?' The word 'person' comes from the Latin word 'persona,' which referred to the masks worn by actors, which they would project sound through to carry their voice out into the audience. When they played a different character they would put on a new mask. Therefore, the 'person' is the mask or the role you're playing."

He then went on to joke that everyone who wants to be a real person is really just learning how to be a genuine fake. Recently, I've noticed people in my life saying how they appreciate my persona. While at first I thought it to be negative, it reminded me that I can consciously choose my context at any moment. While most of my life may be lived on autopilot, masks show me that I can actually choose to be serious, silly, or seductive at the snap of my fingers. And so can you.

Ultimately, the goal with masks outlined in my Men's Weekend, that I will not explore in depth here, is to develop one, three dimensional mask. This persona is who you are as a man, and, if you're conscious about developing all aspects of your character, you can become bold, empathetic, and not take yourself, and the world, too seriously all in one. It's called being three-dimensional.

Being a three-dimensional man is something to strive towards because, as you approach any battlefield in your life, you're prepared to effortlessly shift your tone and attitude no matter the context.

Now that we're aware that as men we wear masks, let's explore a few examples of how we use them before getting to the root of how we let them prevent us from being honest about our pain, addictions, and arrows.

We Wear Masks To Provide

Just like how a warrior used his armor to help him be successful on the battlefield, we use our masks to help us be successful in our careers, relationships, and in all the high-stakes scenarios of our lives. For example, when I started my career in sales, I needed to be confident, competent, and honourable in order to be successful. On the days when I hadn't slept well, was emotional because of a breakup, or just wasn't feeling it, I didn't have the luxury to show up grumpy and disheveled on my sales calls.

If I wanted to be professional and represent myself and my company effectively, I needed to show up at my best regardless of how I felt. This is the power of masks. The warrior doesn't get to take a day off just because he's not feeling it today, when the rest of his tribe is rushing into battle. If he didn't put on his armor, pick up his sword, and remember his training, his brothers would die, and later, probably his family too. In the context of modern success, this is where we leverage our masks to make sure, no matter how we feel, we bring forth our best effort.

Before making a call or starting a sales meeting, I would frequently anchor myself to a context I picked up from the *Straight Line Persuasion* audio program: "Sharp as a tack, enthusiastic as hell, and a force to be reckoned with. "It would help me make sure I brought my A-game. This mask helped me and my clients become more successful because it gave both of us confidence.

While it may seem obvious that you'd always want to bring your best, if you observe a lot of men, they wear masks that don't work. You probably remember a high stakes moment of your life where you didn't do a great job controlling your attitude, tone, or context.

In sales, it's common for a sales professional to show up on a client call where their subconscious communication is that they desperately need a sale, that they're impatient with their prospect, or that they're timid and lacking confidence.

None of these masks work effectively in this context. Therefore, you can see how being conscious of how you show up in your professional life, and what mask you decide to wear, will dramatically impact the success of your career. Think of some of the most successful men in the world like Steve Jobs, Elon Musk, or Warren Buffet. Although they likely wouldn't call what they're doing wearing a mask, when they walk on stage to explain their newest product launches or talk to their shareholders, that's what they're doing.

All of the preparation, failures, and wins they've had in their careers led them to the refinement of their mask overtime, putting them in the best position to be successful. Do you think they just went up there and hoped for the best? Or do you think they were intentional about how to deliver their messages? One mistake in that context would cost them and their shareholders hundreds of millions, if not billions, of dollars. Those stages are their battlefields and you can believe that they did everything they could to prepare themselves.

Another useful way to think about masks in the context of success is the game face. Roger Federer, Lebron James, Peyton Manning, and all of your favourite athletes have been developing and refining their game face for decades. Now, when they step on the battlefield, being confident, relaxed, and bulletproof is second nature. This phenomena of using your mask to help you be successful was best demonstrated in the largest comeback in Super Bowl history by Tom Brady and the New England Patriots against the Atlanta Falcons in Super Bowl LI.

The Patriots were down 28-3 after the Falcons scored a touchdown with only 8:31 left in the third quarter. Whether they'd admit it or not, virtually any other player and team would have given up at this point. But not Tom Brady. Brady and the Patriots went on to complete 43 of 62 pass attempts for 466 yards with two touchdowns and one interception. As Iain, who originally shoved his phone in my face to force me to watch the comeback video (thank you) pointed out, the game was on the line on every single play. One mistake and the game was over.

This is where Brady's "tough as nails "and "do whatever it takes" game face he'd developed his entire career separated him from any other player in the game. If he, as the leader of his team, dropped his mask for even a moment to reveal his uncertainty, the game would have been lost. He described the experience in an interview on the Howard Stern recalling how he talked to his teammates: "You can look at that situation and basically quit and say, 'You know, fuck it. We have no shot of winning,' or you can say, as my teammate, Julian Edelman, repeated, 'It's going to be a hell of a story.' "

Maintaining his armor, his mask, or his game face, when all hope seemed lost was the difference between a blowout and the greatest comeback in Super Bowl history.

If the punchline wasn't clear enough, masks help men be successful. It's important to build this context before talking about where masks go wrong because masks aren't the problem to why men struggle with their mental health. The problem for men and mental health relating to masks is that we have so many men struggling and no place for them to take their mask off.

WE WEAR MASKS TO PROTECT

In order to illustrate how we use masks to protect us, I will share with you, like Juice WRLD shared with us, my biggest insecurity.

Juice sang:

> **Let's be for real**
> **If it wasn't for the pills, I wouldn't be here**
> **But if I keep taking these pills, I won't be here, yeah**
> **I just told y'all my secret, yeah**
> **It's tearing me to pieces**
> **I really think I need them**
> **I stopped taking the drugs and now the drugs take me**

So let's be for real. At 19, I developed a habit that helped me make progress with my depression; I started going to the gym. This wasn't completely new for me since I was a gymnast and athlete as a boy, but it was novel considering I hadn't felt like exercising in a long time. Only a couple weeks in, I started to feel stronger physically and mentally. In a few months, I felt more confident, I had energy I hadn't experienced since long before my depression, and I actually started smiling again. I was happy for the first time in over a year and hooked like an addict.

I started spending two hours a day, seven days a week in the gym. Every day, I worked harder and harder for six months. With my ego engaged, working harder and harder started to look like lifting heavier and heavier. Then, seven years ago, in 2014, on a sunny Saturday morning, I fucked up. I loaded 225lbs on the bar and planned to do 55 deadlifts for time—in the Crossfit community that means as fast as possible. On the 48th deadlift, the gym's manager interrupted. He asked, "Hey, can you keep it down, man? "The bar's contact with the floor was shaking the gym so he put a black mat underneath the weights for cushioning.

In a rush to finish, I went for the 49th rep when the grip of my left hand slipped. I reached for the bar before it fell, and, as I caught it, pulled upwards. I felt the abdomen under my left rib cage pop out and back in. Because the deadlift is a full body exercise, I also felt my shoulder and back, as well as the muscles in my chest, bicep, rotator cuff, and lats, pull abruptly. Considering the amount of weight I was lifting, I should have cooled down, gone home, and observed my injuries to make some decisions about what to do next. Considering I was lifting with my ego and not my commitment, and was probably in shock, I finished the workout.

That night I layed in my bed crying because my abdomen was pulsating and my back was so tight I could hardly move. I wish that was the end of the story. Two days later, I was back in the gym, lifting again. In only a few moments of unconsciousness, my entire reality changed. I put my body through tremendous trauma and went from feeling like an athlete again to making everyday movements, like bending over, a struggle. As of this writing, seven years later, I cannot do a push up without pain. I can't have sex without pain. And even sitting here, writing in my hermit shack on the hill of San Marcos, Guatemala, has my back barking at me in discomfort.

My body is my greatest source of insecurity. And because of that, just like Juice WRLD, I've always been wearing a mask.

In High school, my Mask was so convincing that I was addicted to smoking weed, I skipped class, and felt depressed for months before my parents even said a word. I didn't want others to worry and so I lied that I was okay. Now, I wear a mask to hide my shame and insecurity from the world to protect myself from being hurt even further.

Like we uncovered in Chapter 1, the way I related to my mental health had me denying, deflecting, and avoiding my pain instead of being honest with myself and the world about how I felt. You do this too. And so do men all over the world. In the same way that warriors would wear armor to protect themselves from enemy attacks, we wear our armor to protect our ego, our pride, and our illusion of masculinity.

Maybe you didn't get the promotion at work that you worked your ass off for, so you wear a mask and act like it wasn't that important to you anyways. Or maybe you were dumped by the girl of your dreams so you pretend you didn't like her that much. Or maybe you just lost a son, or a sister, or a loved one in a tragic accident, and you want to be the rock for your family so you use your mask to reassure them that everythings okay. No matter the reason, when men take arrows on the battlefields of their lives, they put on masks to prevent others from seeing their pain and to protect themselves from the possibility of deeper wounds.

I remember how hard I tried to not let my injuries define me. I spent thousands of dollars on chiropractors, physiotherapists, personal training and more. I tried popular workout methodologies, like Original Strength, Kinstretch, Functional Range Conditioning and even my own weird Frankenstein programs of everything mixed together. I would be at the gym lifting 5lbs dumbbells watching my friends from the office bench pressing together feeling like I'd never make progress.

One day out of the blue, I got a group Slack message as a joke from a colleague with a picture of a man with a disfigured body and shrunken biceps with the note, "I found Jonathan's body double. "That was a major low for me. For men, we're bombarded with messages about masculinity and how we're supposed to be strong, tough, and powerful. I couldn't help but look in the mirror and tell myself that I wasn't a man.

After that day, I shoved the mask I was wearing to protect myself from the world even tighter and started doing my daily mobility program, not in the gym, but at home or in a secluded part of the local park. We didn't have an apartment big enough for working out inside and so I spent many hours stretching or practicing a movement I found on YouTube outside in the rain. While I've shared with you part of my story, this is not a space for me to be completely mask down.

There's more to my pain and more to my arrows. But because this is a public forum and not the confines of a confidential space, I will share what is appropriate here, given the context, and the rest in private with my men's team. At this point, I started using a secondary strategy common to men who use masks to protect themselves. I learned to double down on the mask that was working so as to draw attention away from the areas of my life I wanted to hide.

When I hurt my body, I started focusing more on my career to cover it up. By focusing on being more and more successful in business and in my social impact, I was able to hide more effectively the insecurities of my physical health. Mentor and Relationship Coach Steve Richmond describes using masks in this way for protection like the street artist who asks you to guess which shell has a ball underneath it. He puts the ball under a shell and then uses sleight of hand to confuse you where it is. He makes you pay attention to the wrong one so that, when you guess incorrectly, he takes your money.

This is another way men use masks to protect them. Oftentimes, when we get the news that someone killed themselves, we are completely shocked. While most exterior signs pointed to a great life, they were, in fact, wearing a highly effective mask to protect those they loved from worrying, and themselves from having to face their pain head on. I've spoken to dozens of parents who've lost children to suicide and many couldn't believe it. Even those people who were closest, who loved them most, and who knew them best, were convinced by the mask worn by these young people for protection.

This is true for me and also again for Juice WRLD in his music career. His music has been downloaded billions of times but, in his song *Bad Energy*, he sings:

> **In the studio pourin' out my feelings**
> **Can't explain this feeling**
> **Kinda feels like I'm losing**
> **Even though I'm winning**

Juice WRLD acknowledged that from all exterior and traditional metrics of success, he was winning. In fact, with over 30 million active monthly listeners on Spotify alone, Juice WRLD is one of the most successful artists of all time. But that doesn't account for the fact that he's dead. The same goes for Avicii, Kurt Cobain, Chester Bennington, Robin Williams, Mac Miller and hundreds more traditionally successful men who've killed themselves.

Most men would have looked at their lives from the outside and given anything to trade places with them. The problem is that, inside, all of these men were suffering. Instead of being able to address their mental health challenges, they doubled down on their mask of success, which protected them from facing their deepest wounds and acted as a decoy for those who could have helped.

Circle Up

"The important thing to remember, "Iain always reminds me, "is that any tool used for good, can also be used for evil. The same hammer that builds the orphanage is the same hammer that murders the orphans. "Masks are great on the battlefield, but are designed to be taken off when you enter a safe space. When a warrior returned to camp after battle, he wouldn't leave his armor on. He'd take it off. He would observe his wounds and address any damage that needed healing with his brothers in arms.

The problem modern men face is that, unlike our warrior ancestors, we don't have any spaces where we feel the safety needed to go mask down.

So, how do so many men get away with their mental health struggle without even the people closest to them being able to do anything about it? The fundamental reason at the root of our crisis is that our context about men's mental health doesn't work. It has men convinced that they're crazy, weak, or less of a man for battling depression, experiencing anxiety, or struggling with their mental health.

This is why we struggle in silence.

This is why conversations about men's mental health and masculinity are riddled with stigma.

And this is why, instead of asking for help, we put on our mask to protect those around us and ourselves.

As a result of the current mental health context we hold to be true, that men who struggle are viewed as weak, we haven't invested nearly enough resources and energy into developing spaces for men that are confidential and where they feel safe to take off their masks. We haven't carried on the legacy of the warrior who embodied empowered masculinity and taught young men to build relationships based on mutual trust and respect. Instead of teaching men to acknowledge the arrows and trauma they experience in their lives, we've been teaching them to get on with life and "man up. "

Choosing to perpetuate the "man up "motto, is how the hammer that builds the orphanage is now responsible for murdering it's orphans.

What to do about all of this is not easy work. Jack.org is an organization paving the way in the youth mental health space, helping young people to change the way they think, feel, and talk about their mental health. And while we can do the same for men, instead of working with a dozen years of unconscious programming like with teenagers, with men, we're working with multiple decades and oftentimes fifty plus years of "man up "thinking and acting.

In order for a lasting positive impact to be realized, we need commitment. It takes commitment to set aside ego and honour the truth of your struggles, addictions, and arrows. It takes commitment to trust other men and develop masculine relationships. And it takes commitment to Circle Up, when for so long we've been convinced we need to man up.

Unlike a friendship where most of the shared experiences are fun and exciting, finding masculine relationships that you can count on are only tested when you need to have an uncomfortable conversation, when you see a man in your life falling into the basement and you need to take a stand for them, or when you've taken an arrow on the battlefield of your life, are struggling, and need a man you trust to call for help.

It's easy to have someone's back when you're both experiencing positive emotions. But that's not commitment. And It's easy to be there for someone when the sea is calm, your sails are full of wind, and the sun is shining brightly. But that's not commitment, either. True commitment, that which transcends the word, means we're in this together, come hell or high water. Commitment is tested when the mood is sour. Commitment means doing what you said you would do long after the mood you said it in has left you. And lastly, it communicates, "Man, You know I got you, no matter what. "☯[9]

The "why "of why we struggle is our man up context. The "how "of how we get away with it is that we wear masks to convince the world we're okay even though we're addicted and suffering. And the "what " of what to do about all of this insight is the purpose of chapter three. "Man, You Know I Got You "*is* the essence of the Circle Up philosophy and the final puzzle piece in shifting an entire generation's way of thinking, feeling, and acting on men's mental health.

I invite you to read-on so as to embody that philosophy yourself and be part of the change you want to see in the world for men and for our mental health.

Circle Up!

British Columbia, Canada - July 2020

Chapter Summary

Men struggle desperately with addiction, mental health, and suicide often without even their closest friends and family knowing before it's too late. How is that? It's because we tell you we're fine, but we're lying—we just don't want you to worry. We take all our feelings and hide them because we don't want anyone to hurt us. As warriors, we wear masks. But as warriors who use masks for protection and success, we need to learn where and with whom it's safe to take them off before it's too late.

---

9 ☯ **Philosophy Footnote:** *"A smooth sea never made a skilled sailor." - Franklin D. Roosevelt*

Resource Summary

Stay close to the resources, quotes, and thinkers you resonated most with in this chapter. Pay attention to what speaks to your heart. If you said to yourself, "I should check that out, "take action immediately.

Wishing Well - Legends Never Die - Juice WRLD

1. **Men's Weekend - Sterling-institute.com - Justin Sterling**
2. **Out of your mind - Audible.com - Alan Watts**
3. **The Greatest Comeback in Football History - You-Tube - Tom Brady**
4. **Bad Energy - Legends Never Die - Juice WRLD**

Self Reflection Opportunity

Once complete, move these notes to your phone. This will serve to summarize what you have learned, as well as ensure the resources, quotes, and ideas you personally resonated with most, are available at your fingertips.

Key points to remember (fill in here):

Where in my life do I wear a mask successfully? What is it about this mask that works?

Where in my life do I wear a mask that says "I'm fine" but I'm not? In this circumstance, what am I protecting myself from?

Do I have a masculine environment in my life that is 100% confidential to take my mask off?

CHAPTER THREE:

WHAT TO DO ABOUT THE MEN'S MENTAL HEALTH CRISIS

"The wound is the place where the light enters you"
Rumi

ANGEL NOAH

In the winter of 2019, I stood beside my brother in his freezing DIY woodworking shop to plan an important project. In less than four months, he and his fiancée were expecting their first baby. Together, Adam and I began working on the crib that their son would soon sleep in. Over the course of the next few months, they had a baby shower, painted the baby's room, and began brainstorming names for their bundle of joy.

Then, the Coronavirus Pandemic quickly changed the world's landscape. The birth date was approaching, but with new social distancing protocols rolled out in Canada and Globally, it didn't look like we'd be able to join Adam and Laura in the hospital for one of the most important days of their lives. I remember it like it was yesterday. I got a call from Adam the night before the birth, "Hey man, just wanted to let you know we're heading to the hospital. It's time."

I felt a cocktail of nervous excitement mixed with hope. Excitement, because the final tenet on my men's team code of honour is "Be an example for children "and I was to be a first time uncle. And hope, because in a time when the world had never been darker and more divided, this new life, this new light, would bring our family closer together than ever before. Knowing I'd wake up the next day with my first nephew, I fell asleep with a big smile on my face and in my heart.

At the time, Iain and I had been living in a cramped and cold basement apartment where we had to duck to get into our rooms. So, when the rest of the world was working from home to prevent the spread of Coronavirus, the two of us, unwilling to spend all day in those conditions, walked the 300 meter commute and shared the office space designed for 200+ employees alone. That morning, I sent Adam a text from my desk saying, “Sending love, man. Can you update me as soon as things progress? Love you so much <3. ”

I looked up from my phone to see the sun warmly shining through the window behind me and Iain sitting across the room reading *The Denial of Death* by Ernest Beckart. It was 10:23 a.m. when I got the phone call from Adam. “Hey, man, ”I could hear him choking up as he spoke, “there was a complication with the birth. ”He then told me that, when the doctors tried to deliver the baby, he got stuck in the birth canal.

Their equipment told them his breathing stopped, so to get him out faster, they performed an emergency C-section. He was unresponsive and so they gave him CPR. The doctors, who were able to kickstart his heart, quickly moved him to intensive care. Adam told me that they wouldn't have any information for us about his health until they did an MRI at Sick Kids Hospital later in the week.

Of all of the possibilities I'd dreamt of the night before, I never imagined our call going this way. My brother, ready and excited to be a father, and Laura, bravely and enthusiastically carrying their child for almost a year, were now to wait a full week in helpless anxiety of the news to come. Unable to go to the hospital or hold each other, our whole family wept that day for the inexplicable pain Laura and Adam were experiencing. I felt numb.

Adam sent me a picture from the intensive care unit so our family could see baby Noah for the first time. It was crystal clear to me that my nephew was, and is, a certified fucking stud.

Five days later, the MRI showed major brain damage. The blind faith we had clung to to be there for Adam and Laura evaporated. The doctor made it clear that Noah would never walk, talk, or ever experience the beauty our world has to offer. With that, the decision was made to take him off life support and bring him home where we could make him as comfortable as possible, surrounded by his friends and family, in the last days of his life.

A couple of days later, I drove from the city to hold Noah and sing him my favourite songs on the guitar. I remember his eyes flickered as I played "Hey Maria "by Klangarussell - Elderbrook Remix and sang,

> **"All these years go by**
> **You roll by my side**
> **Go ahead, run that line**
> **You know I got you, yeah"**

Although Laura told me he liked my voice, I'm sure he would have told me to cut it out if he could have. I'll never forget the helplessness I felt knowing there was nothing I could do to make things better for Adam, Laura, or Noah. All I could do was hold him, love him, and whisper, "You know I got you. "Often when we experience tragedy, our immediate response is to look for a solution and pursue it with all of our energy. On that day, there were no solutions, only surrender.

In less than a week, Noah passed. There are no words to describe the massive spears that had just pierced and lodged themselves firmly inside of Adam and Laura. It's moments like these, where our friends and families take arrows on the battlefield of life, that we're forced to take a step back, pull our eyes off our email and the business of day-to-day life, and remember what is important: love.

MAN, YOU KNOW I GOT YOU

The "why "of why we struggle is a "man up "context that doesn't serve our men in the way it's being communicated or perceived. The "how "of how we get away with it is that we wear masks to convince the world we're okay even though we're not. And the "what "of what to do about all of this insight, derived from the last decade of paying attention to my own mental health, is best encapsulated in the months that followed Noah's death.

After Noah died, I defaulted to holding onto my grief and wearing my mask that everything was okay. Even after all these years of mental health advocacy, I still let the inherited context around mental health and masculinity influence my actions. I didn't want to admit that I needed help. Most importantly I wanted to be a rock for my family in a time of tragedy.

Less than two weeks later, I remember being called out by one of the experienced men on my men's team for looking miserable. He noticed I wasn't being myself and so the team "burned the agenda " for our meeting and created the space for me to cry and scream out on Zoom. I had confronted arrows with my men in the past, but always in person, and never of this severity. Zoom didn't seem to be enough. Leaving that meeting, I felt lethargic and frustrated. Over the next couple weeks, I tried to focus on my career and even women to distract me, but every day I felt more and more drained.

I spent dozens of hours walking through the forest, listening to my favourite music, and trying all of my typical self-care routines, but it wasn't helping. Something was missing. Like most men when they experience loss or tragedy, I hadn't confronted my arrow. Noah's death was slowly pulling me into the basement. I started smoking weed again every day. I was frustrated and pissed off at the world. And my mood felt like a big dark cloud following me everywhere I went.

One day, Iain mentioned that he'd noticed I hadn't been myself recently. He told me that he cared and asked what he could do to be there for me. We made a plan that, the next day, we would curate a list of our favourite songs and dance together in our favourite park. The next morning, we configured our playlist, ate a microdose of psilocybin mushrooms and a weed edible, and set off for our mini adventure. At the time, most of High Park's trails were off limits because of the Pandemic, so we took an unmarked path into the bush.

We followed it for about fifteen minutes, half walking, half dancing, our headphones synced playing our favourite songs the whole way. When we reached a massive tree, we both threw down our bags and started clearing away the sticks and debris to make room to dance. I remember the first song to play on that makeshift forest dance floor was the deep menacing vocals and booming techno house of Adam Beyers *Going Down*. Instantly, like we had on hundreds of dance floors before the Pandemic, we became theatrical and silly.

Iain started spinning in place so I used my hands from five feet away to twirl him faster or slower, higher and then lower, and we burst out into laughter. Another epic song, *Lost Souls* the AVIRA remix, came on as we continued to dance hard and shout at the trees and the birds like idiots. It was shenanigans at it's finest.

Finally, as if destiny brought me to this moment, the pace slowed and the playlist transitioned to one of my personal favourite artists, Ash. I saw Iain stop in his place, close his eyes and slowly sway to the guitar and piano of Ash's song *Beausoleil,* so I followed his lead.

The second I closed my eyes, I thought of Noah. I could see him lying limp in my arms, the only movement the flickering of his eyes. I could feel the softness of his skin and the fuzzy toy bunny that accompanied him. I could hear every desperate breath his tiny body could muster and knew that anyone of them could be his last. I thought about how unfair it all seemed. I thought of my sister and my parents. And I thought about Adam and Laura and about how all I wanted was to be there for them and tell them it would all be okay.

A tear fell. Then another. I focused again on the music as the climax of Ash's guitar hit and the flood gates opened. Within seconds, Iain's hand was on my shoulder and without needing words he nodded a look that said, "You know I've got you. "He hugged me and I felt all of the apprehension and barriers I'd put up, even with my best friend in the whole world, vanish.

What wasn't possible through Zoom, even though well intentioned, was achieved that day. I wept for the first time since Noah passed and it was one of the most cathartic moments of my life. The safe space Iain created gave me the opportunity to take off the mask I'd been wearing and feel the grief that I'd been pushing away ☯[10].

Crying for the loss and acknowledging the pain that my family went through doesn't make me less of a man. It makes me human.

It's our struggle, our challenge, and our arrows that unite us. Being there for each other when the easy thing to do is hide, confronting the pain when all we want to do is drown it out, and pulling out our arrows when every instinct is screaming to numb ourselves, is the uncomfortable truth of what to do about the men's mental health crisis. That experience, along with the masculine care I've received over the years from my dad and countless other men, has changed how I think, feel, and act on my mental health forever.

I pulled out my arrow that day because of Iain's care for me. It doesn't mean I never feel sad about Noah or that I don't cry when I think about him and our loss. It just means that I've given his life, and his death, new meaning. Noah taught us that, although pain is inevitable, suffering is a choice. He reminded us of how fleeting this life can be. And that all we really have, and all that really matters, is our commitment to loving each other.

Noah was, and is, loved deeply. His life was a gift and brought our family closer together than ever before. Because of him, I *will* be an example for children. I will laugh and love and try to live every day of this precious life to its fullest. And I will hold his memory close to my heart.

---

10 ☯ **Philosophy Footnote:** ♥ - *Iain Gabriel*

This book and the work I do with men's mental health is dedicated to you, buddy. ☯[11] It's also dedicated to you Adam, and to you, Laura. No one should have to endure what you have endured. Yet you have. Noah's light shines with us now. That's forever in our hearts. The whole family has got your back, no matter what. We love you.

If I had to boil down the Circle Up philosophy on men's mental health and masculine care in only a few carefully selected words, it would read, "Man, you know I got you."

The words are just a symbol. The meaning, feeling, and promise behind the words are what matters. The Circle Up philosophy, which I also believe to be the "what "in the "what do we do "about our men's mental health crisis, is to ensure every man knows that they're not alone. It's the same feeling my dad gave me when I was struggling in High School. It's the feeling Iain gave me that day in High Park, and through every hardship we've overcome together as best friends. It's the feeling of commitment, where you know without a shadow of a doubt, your brothers have your back. That no matter how gripped you are by addiction right now, how deep the wounds of your arrows, and how hopeless your situation may seem, you are never alone. ☯[12]

So what do we need to do in regards to men and their mental health?

We need to help them not only read the words, but to embrace and embody the philosophy. As we discovered in chapter one, the addictions we use to cope with, the masks we wear to protect ourselves, and the silence of our struggle are just the fruits, not the roots of the problem.

In order to have men embrace a new way of feeling about masculinity, and adopt the patterns of behaviour that will ultimately lead them to positive mental health outcomes, happier families, and thriving communities, we need to begin at the source: our thinking.

---

11 ☯ **Philosophy Footnote:** *"I will not say not to cry, for not all tears are an evil."* **- Gandalf**
"Nor is grief in general an evil. Grief is a revelation of love." **- Iain Gabriel**

12 ☯ **Philosophy Footnote:** *"The wound is where the light enters you."* **- Rumi**

Designing A New Future For Men And For Mental Health

It's taken me ten years to read the books, listen to the audio programs, and collect the experiences necessary to rewire my thinking about my mental health. I would never have been able to take off my mask and weep in Iain's arms with the way we have been wired to think about masculinity and masculine relationships. The balance of this chapter, and this book, is dedicated to communicating a new way of thinking.

The final infinity stone for the Circle Up philosophy came in late 2019, only months before the global Coronavirus Pandemic and our loss of Angel Noah.

I had just walked into the last of three courses of Landmark International's Curriculum For Living, the Self Expression and Leadership Program. Here, they promised to teach us to rewire our beliefs and create a new future from what they called "possibility." And it worked. The over 100 participants in my cohort were to meet for twelve hours once a month, for four months. Additionally, we met every single Monday night for three more hours. We took on this massive commitment because we were given the opportunity to be coached on designing a community service project that would make a difference for our community of choice.☯[13]

Fran, our seminar leader, began by asking us, "What frustrates you about the world and who needs your leadership? "She also asked, "What challenge are they facing? "Why should we do anything about it? And "why should we act now? "This process is the practical aspect of Carl Jung's idea of making the unconscious conscious. Or what Jim Rohn described as learning to set a better sail. It's also the same work that men like Joe Dispensa and James Clear are teaching and using that are changing the world. Together, we will use men's mental

13 ☯ **Philosophy Footnote:** *"Lucy in the sky with diamonds." - The Beatles*

health and Circle Up as an example so you can apply this process to your own life. ☯[14]

First, as you've already seen, we start with a case for action. Why change at all, and what challenges are you facing? Note the additional spaces below. If you don't already have a pen, grab one. This is where you have an opportunity for introspection and awareness. Think of an area in your life (mariage, academics, physical health, finances, etc.) you'd like to address and take advantage of this exercise to live based on a vision for the future instead of your probable almost-certain future if you don't change.

1. **Case For Action**

The case for action describes the current state of affairs. What challenges are you facing?

MEN'S MENTAL HEALTH

Men struggle alone using strategies to cope like sex and drugs
Globally, every minute, a man dies by suicide
75% of suicides in Canada are men

YOUR TURN

Q: Describe an area of your life that you want to progress. What challenges are you facing?

-
-
-

They asked us to *really* feel. "If there's no emotion, "they said, "you will never change your thinking. "So late into the evening of our first 12-hour seminar day, I remember sitting on the floor thinking about all the men we'd loved and lost.

---

14 ☯ **Philosophy Footnote:** *"Carl Jung said, 'We cannot change anything that we do not accept,' so it is important to be honest with ourselves and where we're currently at so that we effectively go where we want. The first step in getting somewhere isn't figuring out where you're going, but figuring out where you are." - Iain Gabriel*

I thought about Dean Rhyno. I thought about an incredible young man from my hometown, Randy Bagg. Of Iain and our buddy Mike's dads, Ren Gabriel and Pete Milewski. I thought of Eric Windeler's son, Jack Windeler. And I thought about their families and how much suffering they must have gone through. I was struck with sadness.

As I held the faces of these men in my mind's eye, I suddenly saw again the image of my dad throwing the bucket of water on me as a teenager. Of him sitting with me on my drenched bed. Him holding me and reminding me that I wasn't alone. I had the overwhelming feeling in that moment that, no matter what, the people in my life had my back. ☯[15]

Almost immediately, things were different. All of my uncertainty about how to create the community project vanished. *If men who were struggling could get the idea into their minds of Circle Up instead of man up,* I thought, *that could be the future.* The memory of my dad's gift to me transformed my sadness, uncertainty, and doubt, into a desire to act. I once again became present to the excitement of the participants in the room, and, for a last time, held the image in my mind of all the men in our lives that we'd loved and lost, and started writing what a different future could look like. It would be their legacy.

2. Inherited Context

The next step is to bring into your awareness the unconscious beliefs that are producing your current results. It's only by making them conscious, as Jung suggested, that we're able to choose a new fate.

What do you believe about yourself or the world that is driving these current results in your life?

15 ☯ **Philosophy Footnote:** *"You know we got you." - Iain Gabriel*

MEN'S MENTAL HEALTH

Only crazy people have issues with their mental health
Struggling with my mental health makes me weak and less of a man
I need to "man up" when I'm stressed or struggling with my mental health

YOUR TURN

Q: What beliefs about yourself and the world are responsible for these problems in your life?

-
-
-

3. Probable Almost Certain Future

The next step to rewire your thinking is to consider the probable almost-certain future if you do nothing about it. The key here, again, is to fully feel the emotions associated with your probable almost-certain future.

When you imagine how your life will turn out if you don't change, does it make you feel angry? Do you feel hopeless? Do you feel ashamed?

Whatever the feeling, visualize the probable almost-certain future and go deeply into those feelings. For until the pain of staying the same is greater than the pain of change, you will remain bound.

Men's Mental Health

- Men will distrust each other, suffer in silence, and feel separate from the world
- Men will become more and more addicted to short term pain relief and turn to sex and drugs to cope with their mental health
- Men will will hide their pain with masks and our families and communities will continue to be destroyed as globally a man kills himself every minute

Your Turn

Q: What is the probable almost-certain future for you if you don't change this area of your life?

4.1 Creating Possibility (actions, feelings, people, and places)

Creating possibility is the final step in rewiring your beliefs.

How would you need to look at the world, and how would you need to look at yourself, in order to create a different outcome?

Bring forth in your mind's eye your vision for your future.

What does it look like? What are you doing? Who are you with? What habits do you practice? Who are you being? What feelings are associated with this new life? Do you feel pride? Do you feel more love and energy? Do you feel gratitude?

The key to calling this new future towards you is to feel those emotions now. Imagine your new future vividly and linger in the emotion of that new life as long as possible.

MEN'S MENTAL HEALTH

Men develop masculine relationships that are built on trust, honour, and a commitment to each other's well being and success
Men come together in confidential spaces where they share the challenges of their lives, discover and dissolve the barriers holding them back, and are held accountable to stepping into that new vision for the future
Men know how and where to take off their mask and ask for help even when it's uncomfortable, painful, or overwhelming

YOUR TURN

Q: What is the vision for your future? Do not see this as an intellectual exercise. Use this as a workbook and something you will come back to, improve over time, and implement. Outline your new future in the greatest detail possible. If you run out of space, transfer these notes to a journal or a note on your phone.

-
-
-

4.2 Creating Possibility (thoughts and beliefs)

Q: Finally, what would you have to believe about yourself, or the world, to make that vision of the future come to fruition? In other words, what context would serve you best? What intentional set of the sail can you embody, and make decisions from, that actualize that vision you've created for yourself?

MEN'S MENTAL HEALTH

> **Every man has mental health and no man struggles alone. Don't man up, Circle Up.**

YOUR TURN

Q: What beliefs about yourself, or the world, will best serve you in calling into existence your new life?

-

If you have followed along up to this point (I encourage you to go back if you haven't), you now have a mantra and personal philosophy that will serve you in creating a new life. You no longer need to be limited by memories of the past, your current circumstances, or of your unconscious and inherited beliefs.

That process demonstrated your leadership, self-expression, and power to consciously create the lens in which you look at the world. That lens, as we described earlier, is the difference in how your life turns out. To repeat Jim Rohn one more time, that lens is the sail on your sailboat. And the reason it's so important is because it's not what happens to you that determines the destination in your life, it's what you do about what happens. What happens, happens to everyone.

How you look at it, interpret it, and what you do or do not do about it, makes all the difference.

Key Point: You cannot change the destination of your life overnight, but you can change the direction.

It took your whole life to think what you think, believe what you believe, and choose the actions you take on a daily basis. Therefore, reading this chapter and completing the above exercises are not enough to alter your thoughts instantaneously. The point of this chapter is to help you introspect, gain awareness about your thoughts and life, and to take the first step.

This is where Jim Roh's idea that, "You cannot change the destination of your life overnight, but you can change the direction "applies practically. If you took this process seriously and created a new possibility for your life, you may very well have changed your direction. Your destination, however, will be determined only through the disciplined application of choosing your new life day in and day out.

In order to further facilitate this process, I recommend a complementary practice created by neuroscientist Dr. Joe Dispenza.

1. **Search Joe's free morning meditation on YouTube or Spotify**
2. **Meditate on the vision for your future every day for thirty days**

If that sounds too daunting, consider giving it a shot at least one time. ☯[16] This guided meditation will take the uncertainty out of making the unconscious conscious. Further, the importance of this daily practice cannot be overemphasized. The brain is designed to take the path of least resistance and repeat habits that you've developed over time. Although it's my hope that my writing is inspirational and gets you started, if you do not reinforce through daily visualization, the new life you desire, and the choices that person would make

16 ☯ **Philosophy Footnote:** *"If you had one shot, or one opportunity, to seize everything you ever wanted in one moment Would you capture it or just let it slip?" - Eminem*

daily, you will find yourself quickly falling back into your old ways of thinking and being.

Following these guided meditations will have you engaged in the discipline of designing your new life, daily. If you're truly committed to your thriving mental health, this is the most well organized resource I've found in transformation. As Joe encourages in his guided morning meditation, "This is your experiment with destiny."

Circle Up

With the outline of our Landmark project completed, they began handing out sheets of paper called "weekly action plans "and asked us to start making commitments. Most of them were extremely uncomfortable. The important ones almost always are. While I was originally afraid that my friends wouldn't care about this work, what I found was everyone that said yes had their own mental health journey and reasons for wanting to participate. Soon, we found that there were dozens of men who were ready to have this conversation and be part of creating a better future for themselves, their families, and their communities.

On February 28th, 2020, with a blizzard hitting the city of Toronto, thirty men gathered around a massive bonfire on the lakeshore to normalize a conversation about men's mental health. It was the official beginning of Circle Up. That day, and over the next eight weeks, we did the work of developing empowered masculine relationships based on confidentiality, mutual respect, and trust. We learned about masks, arrows, addictions, and what to do about them. My role in the overall mission, hardly more than a spark.

Once men were meeting virtually to have these conversations, one leader after another found Circle Up and began to transform it into what it is today. They quickly formed a new leadership team with decades of experience to match our pace of growth. Soon enough, these men (you know who you are) gave Circle Up wings with their energy and enthusiasm and took the idea that no man is alone and turned it into a global movement for men's mental health and empowered masculinity. Circle Up is the future of man up. With now over a hundred men from all over the world graduating from our 10-week men's circle, Circle Up is beginning to have a global impact.

The themes we explored in these first three chapters are just the tip of the iceberg of what we practice and teach. We began this journey with the promise of exposing some of the major reasons why men struggle, how they get away with it, and what to do about it. I believe we've accomplished that goal. With the purest of intentions, I hope we've also accomplished a secondary goal, to nudge you along the path of your own personal development.

One of my favourite Rumi quotes reads, "Yesterday I was clever, so I wanted to change the world. Today, I am wise, so I am changing myself."

As men who want to be part of leading others to honour their mental health and come together to heal, we'd best begin by healing ourselves.

Once you become the type of man who changes your thinking from "man up "to "Circle Up "and from "struggling makes you weak "to "you know I got you, "you give every man in your life the permission to do the same. Just like no one can do your push ups for you, no one can do the work of changing the way you think, feel, and act on your mental health but yourself. These three first chapters of why, how, and what, are like the foundation of a house. Before you begin adding drywall, constructing bathrooms, and adding a roof, you first need to take the time to carefully and meticulously ensure that the foundation is secure.

Building your dream home on a foundation of sand is delusional and a recipe for frustration. Therefore, what you just did, by being honest about your current beliefs, thinking, and life, and then reimagining a future from possibility instead of from your memories of the past, was doing the work of digging a new foundation. The balance of this book is about constructing that new life.

Taking off your mask and holding a mirror up to your face to see the truth, imperfections and all, takes tremendous courage. You and only you hold the key to your better future. This is the process. You are on the path. My encouragement is to leverage that strength and momentum in the direction of your new life, remembering that you're not on this path of life change alone, you know we got you. ☯[17]

Circle Up!

Santa Teresa, Costa Rica - February 2021

17 ☯ **Philosophy Footnote:** *"Life, we don't have to figure it out alone." - Mark Nguyen*

Chapter Summary

Up to this point, men have been conditioned to struggle alone, hide their pain, and man up. This is not the way. If we continue to perpetuate this level of thinking, we can only create more of the same results. So how do we create new possibilities for men, their families, and our communities? A new future requires a new vision. For men to thrive, we need to stop thinking man up and start thinking Circle Up. Once we personally become the type of men who change our thinking from "man up "to "circle up "and from "struggling makes you weak "to "you know I got you, "we give every man in our lives the permission to do the same. Planting new seeds will create a radically new harvest.

Resource Summary

Stay close to the resources, quotes, and thinkers you resonated most with in this chapter. Pay attention to what speaks to your heart. If you said to yourself, "I should check that out, "take action immediately.

1. Denial Of Death - Ernest Becker
2. Hey Maria - Elderbrook Remix
3. Going Down - Adam Beyer
4. Lost Souls - AVIRA Remix
5. Beausoleil - Ash
6. Self-Expression and Leadership Course - Curriculum For Living - Landmark Worldwide
7. Morning Meditation - Spotify / YouTube - Joe Dispenza

Self-Reflection Opportunity

Once complete, move these notes to your phone. This will serve to summarize what you have learned, as well as ensure the resources, quotes, and ideas you personally resonated with most.

Key points to remember (fill in here):

What is one idea from this chapter that will help me "set a better sail" in my own personal philosophy?

CHAPTER FOUR:

SELF-CARE: AN ACT OF SELF-LESSNESS

"I will take care of me, so that I can take care of you, if you would please take care of you, so that you can take care of me."

Jim Rohn

FOUNDATIONS FIRST, CONSTRUCTION SECOND

There is no one I've learned more about changing the way we think, feel, and act on mental health than from Eric Windeler and the team at Jack.org. While working full-time in software sales, I applied another of Jim Rohn's fundamental teachings and decided to "Work harder on myself than I did on my job. "In order to improve my sales, I joined a local Toastmasters group committed to improving leadership and communication skills. It turned out, Jim was right. The best investment I could make was one in myself.

When I walked into the room at CSI Pitchmasters, I was blown away at their energy and enthusiasm for personal development. I was home. Every week, we practiced prepared speeches and impromptu presentations. Even though I didn't feel ready, I was encouraged to give my first speech a try by Iain who reminded me, "Anything that's worth being good at is worth being bad at first. "After the meeting, a woman named Karen came up to me and said, "I know some young people who could benefit from that story. "She introduced me to another woman who opened more doors, and, all of a sudden, I had given a dozen free speeches regarding mental health that year.

Many months and many opportunities for impact later, I found myself sharing the stage with Eric Windeler. I was speaking on behalf of one of the most reputable organizations in mental health at the time, Healthy Minds Canada, and was moved to tears from what Eric shared about his son, Jack, and his suicide as a first year student at Queens University. In his speech, he spoke about the moment the Police Officer broke the news to him and his family, and how it felt like a cluster bomb had gone off.

He described the rollercoaster they went through, and how, if a tragedy like this could happen to them, it could happen to anyone. The more he learned about mental health, the more he found out he was right. He and his wife Sandra found that suicide had become the #1 related health cause of death for young people in Canada. So Eric quickly decided to set aside his business interests to be part of changing the way Canadian's looked at, and acted upon, their mental health. ☯[18]

Jack.org, the organization he founded along with his wife and family, had quickly transformed from a youth outreach project, partnered with Kids Help Phone, to Canada's largest youth mental health charity. In less than two years, they shifted their model from talking at students, to including them in the conversation. It worked. They successfully developed a peer-to-peer model that empowered young people to develop leadership and advocacy skills. Today, there are over 2,500 youth leaders across Canada who give Jack Talks, lead Jack Chapters, and organize community events committed to normalizing help-seeking behaviours and mental health advocacy.

No man, besides my own father's actions, have inspired me more to make a contribution in the field of mental health than Eric. In my eyes, he and his family are the truest definition of resilience. He is

---

18 ☯ **Philosophy Footnote:** *"Be the change you wish to see in the world." - Gandhi*

living proof of the truth of Jim Rohn's words, "It's not what happens, it's what you do about what happens that determines your future." They have turned what is no doubt the most difficult thing to ever happen to a family into a movement that has forever made a positive impact on the world.

Furthermore, I have yet to personally find a better leadership development opportunity available to young people in Canada interested in mental health. My three years volunteering with Jack.org brought me to schools all across Canada, to share my lived experiences and relate with students. They introduced me to hundreds of new friends and leaders, empowered my voice, and have been instrumental in shaping me to become the type of person that can, and is, making a difference in the world.☯ [19]

Lastly, they are largely responsible for the insight in the balance of this chapter. This is the first of three parts in the construction of your new dream home.☯[20] With the foundation securely in place, we will now layer on top: the walls, the furnishings, and the ceiling of the Circle Up philosophy.

1. **The walls - Self-Care: An Act Of Selflessness**
2. **The furnishing - Masculine Relationships: A Mental Health Revolution**
3. **The ceiling - Off The Couch And Onto The Battlefield + Slaying Dragons**

Grab a hammer and some nails, for the walls must be built. ☯[21]

---

19 ☯ **Philosophy Footnote:** *"In the same way Jonathan is alchemizing his negative mental health experiences into positives through this book and other initiatives, Eric Windler has done a wonderful job of honouring the memory of his son in a way that if he is seeing what is happening, he would be proud. He spurred this thought: 'You get to decide how true the statement 'Everything happens for a reason' is.'" - Iain Gabriel*

20 ☯ **Philosophy Footnote:** *"There are no rules of architecture for castles constructed in the clouds." - G. K. Chesterton*

21 ☯ **Philosophy Footnote:** *"Get the plane ready to enter the clouds." - Iain Gabriel*

Developing A Self-Care Battle Plan

Jack.org taught me that mental health is not a moment in time, but a spectrum that exists throughout your life. There are times when you're thriving and there are times when you're in the basement. So, think of this section as developing a battle plan that addresses your thoughts, feelings, and behaviours.

When you're stressed, what will you do? When you struggle, how will you manage? What habits, resources, and people will you count on to bring you back to feeling at your best? And when you're in a crisis, do you have a plan? Is there someone you trust to call? Most importantly, how can you ensure you'll make that call when you need it most? ☯[22]

Athletes will understand this analogy immediately. When you're on the court and the opposing team changes up their defence, what play will you call? How will you overcome the shift in the context and come out on top? My years as an advocate with Jack.org taught me that mental health is dynamic and ever changing. Therefore, we need a dynamic strategy to help ensure that, no matter the change, we know exactly what to do and when, even when we don't.

In order to develop this battle plan for your life, let's first consider how all of human experience exists on a spectrum. We have a spectrum for light, for radiation, for sound, and these spectrums demonstrate that life isn't black and white, but often somewhere in the gray. Your mental health works in the same way.

This dynamic is crystal clear in the parallel of our physical health. We have a body that we can touch and see. We experience pain like cutting a finger, breaking an arm, or having a heart attack. At any given moment on the spectrum of our physical health, we're somewhere between perfect health and vitality, all the way to disease and chronic illness.

---

22 ☯ **Philosophy Footnote:** *"One of the major determinants of how your life will go is how you emotionally regulate yourself during moments of stress and crisis." - Iain Gabriel*

Because there's not the same taboo or stigma to physical health, over time, we've developed a social and cultural agreement where if you cut your finger, you use a bandaid. If you break your arm, you get a cast. If you jump off a cliff in Guatemala and injure your spine, you call an ambulance (long story short, I'm an idiot). The challenge with mental health is because it's harder to see, we've yet to normalize help-seeking behaviours. We hide these dynamic changes in our mental health instead of having the same "If this, then that "process as we do with physical health.

As a result, instead of practicing self-care and help-seeking behaviours, we now have men all over the world who don't acknowledge when they're stressed or struggling, and protect themselves from the world with their masks. When we feel stress, we don't take five deep breaths or go for a walk. When we're struggling, we don't see a counsellor or join a men's team. And when we're in crisis, we're often so out of control that calling for help is the last thing on our minds.

Until we're able to embrace a new social and cultural context, acknowledging that we all have mental health, the most practical next step in constructing the castle of your dreams is to take responsibility for developing your own plan. A plan that:

1. **Gets you out of your head and back onto the battlefield of your life and**
2. **Prevents you from crossing the chasm between stress and struggle by pausing and getting help before it's too late.**

If This, Then That

When I was a lifeguard in my teenage years, we spent a lot of time learning how to identify a variety of signs and symptoms of physical health struggles. I was trained to deal with everything from the basics of nose bleeds all the way to emergency situations like heart attacks and strokes. Illness and injury was perceived through a spectrum and the severity of the injury would determine what we would do and who we would call for help. The same applies to our mental health.

How, and by who you can be supported, is determined by where you are on the mental health spectrum at any given moment in your life.

HEALTHY AND STRESSED

Imagine you're walking on the pool deck of your local swimming pool. You suddenly slip and scrape your knee. Immediately, you hear a whistle and I'm running over to you like Zach Efron from *Baywatch*. I point out that there's no blood, just a little bruising. At this level of the physical health spectrum, you can take care of yourself. You may be stressed temporarily from falling, but you're healthy enough to quickly get back in the pool after regaining your composure.

Let's apply these same concepts to developing your mental health action plan. When stress impacts your thoughts, feelings, and behaviours, let's say it's an exam period or a particularly busy season at work, we can turn to self-care coping strategies to stay at our best. This is a time when resources like *Atomic Habits* by James Clear become particularly useful. Situations that induce stress act as a "queue, "where if you're not conscious of your habits, it can trigger unwanted decisions and behaviours.

For example, over time, getting an email from your boss may have become your queue to take a cigarette break. Or maybe long hours of studying and cramming for exams becomes your queue to order skip-the-dishes and stuff your face with a full pizza. Often, stress, and our response to it, will determine the direction our lives are taking. If you respond to the daily queues of stress with habits that support you in the direction of becoming the man you've always wanted to be, you'll quickly bounce back to health.

On the other hand, if you continuously choose avoidant behaviours or the path of least resistance to feel good, like sex, porn, drugs, or processed foods in the face of stress, you're more likely to move in the direction of struggle in respect to your mental health. Another useful tip from *Atomic Habits* is to think of these responses to stress as an election system. Every time you choose to act in congruence with the

"If this, then that," actions you will define for yourself below, you're casting a vote for the man you've always wanted to be.

Every time you choose old thinking, old feelings, and your old actions in response to the stress you experience in life, you're casting a vote for your current identity, or worse. I encourage you to implement the ideas in this chapter immediately and allow the votes to build up in the favour of your new vision.

Self-Reflection Opportunity

Note the additional spaces below. If you don't already have a pen, grab one. This entire section is designed to be your opportunity for introspection and awareness. Think of it as being on the court in your life. This is your workbook and something you will come back to in order to improve over time and implement in your life.

1.1 Signs and symptoms of stress

When you experience stress, what does it look like for you? What does it feel like? What change in your experience will act as a que for you to implement your new battle plan?

My example

Restless sleeping at night
Shallow breathing
Anxiety and feeling like other people are judging me or thinking about me negatively
Tension in my neck, shoulders, and upper back
Desire for quick hits of dopamine, especially from social media, weed, and sugar
Showing up late to meetings, calls, and events
Negative self-talk and being over-critical and analyzing all of my decisions
Reduced desire to follow my routines and habits like exercise, healthy eating, and meditation
Late responding to messages, emails, and business opportunities

Your Turn

Q: What are some of the indicators in your life that you're feeling stressed?

1.2 "If this, then that" action plan to stress

My Example

1. **Lay down on the floor and breath deeply for 5-10 minutes relaxing my mind and body**
2. **Go for a walk outside and listen to my favourite music or call someone I love**
3. **Write down three things I'm grateful for and send an appreciation text or video to a friend**

Key Point: Standardize before you optimize.

Doubt kills the warrior and only action can cut through the doubt. Start with the easiest action in response to stress that aligns in the direction of your new life. Eventually, when you have chosen your new life enough, or casted enough votes, you can make your responses to stress progressively more beneficial and elaborate.

When Iain started his meditation habit, for example, he started with five breaths before bed and when he woke up. Those five breaths eventually grew to five, and then ten minutes. And, in a few months, those 10 minutes grew to over 20 minutes a day. ☯ [23]

---

23 ☯ **Philosophy Footnote:** *"On God" - Juice WRLD*
"Jonathan and I allowed this to be a queue to listen to Juice WRLD's 'On God,' and dance around like the fools that we are. Don't take yourself too seriously!" - Iain Gabriel

For myself personally, when I first created my "If this, then that" response to stress, instead of laying down on the floor for ten minutes, I would sit down and take three deep breaths. Eventually, I noticed how much better I felt after only three breaths so I decided to turn it into one minute of laying on the floor. Soon enough, that one minute became a ten minute routine where I lay on the floor, put on some chill music (usually FKJ) and use essential oils like lavender for deeper relaxation. Now, any time I feel stressed or want to take a break from writing, work, or my life, I can just lay down and breathe. Actually, that said, let me do that right now.

YOUR TURN

Q: When I notice that I am stressed I can and I will:

1.
2.
3.

Key Point: "If this, then that" is context dependent.

It's the exception rather than the rule that I will do all three actions on my "If this, then that" action plan in response to stress. Almost always, what I can, and what I will do, when I notice I'm stressed is context dependent. When I felt stressed working in sales at a 200 person company, it was much easier to write down what I was grateful for and or go for a quick walk than it was to lay down on the floor and breathe for ten minutes.

If you're feeling stressed and one of your action items is to go for a walk in nature, but it's minus forty degrees outside or torrential downpouring, use whichever "If this, then that" response to stress that is most appropriate for the context. Even if you have to adapt or modify the positive behaviour you've chosen temporarily, I encourage you to get excited about casting that vote for the man you've always wanted to be. They will quickly add up. ☯[24]

Struggling

I believe it's the acknowledgement of our mental health struggle where we have the greatest opportunity to make a positive impact for ourselves and the world. Imagine, this time, you're swimming towards the wall of the pool and you crash face first into the tiling. Your nose starts to bleed and the lifeguard pulls you into their office to take care of it. He's concerned that you may have hit your head hard enough for a concussion and so he recommends you to be taken to the hospital for a second opinion.

This is assisted care. It's why community resources exist. In the world of physical health, these resources look like lifeguards, paramedics, physicians, personal care workers and hundreds more. These individuals are trained professionals and work to maintain the health and safety of the public. The exact same type of assisted care exists for us when we're struggling with our mental health—we've simply neglected them.

We have family doctors, psychotherapists, counsellors, anonymous help lines, Alcoholics Anonymous, men's circles and more. Our challenge is that, while there's no stigma in going to the physiotherapist for your knee, there's a massive stigma when it comes to seeking help with our mental health. We know now that there's no reason to feel this way. Every man has mental health and the capacity to struggle. Instead of manning up, as our social conditioning has taught us, with our new foundation of thinking, we can Circle Up and ask for help or seek the appropriate resources to support us.

Before considering what to do about our mental health struggles, it's important to know what it looks like. While stress manifests itself differently for every person, struggle is well observed with little variance from person to person. Just like a lifeguard knew what to look

---

24 ☯ **Philosophy Footnote:** *"What's easy to do is also easy not to do... Get excited about your ability to make yourself do the necessary things." - Jim Rohn*

for when someone was having a heart attack, you can do the same thing with the signs and symptoms of mental health struggles.

Reflecting back on chapter one, my men's team refers to mental health struggles synonymously with the idea of being in the basement. Take an inventory of yourself and see if you or any man in your life is currently expressing any of these signs of struggle:

- Negative view of self
- Neglect of physical appearance or hygiene
- A sense of hopelessness for the future
- Self isolation or desire to be alone
- Dodging others attempts at support or contact
- Drastic changes in mood and behaviour
- Substance abuse
- Self-harm
- Suicidal ideation, both thoughts as well as planning

2.1 Signs and symptoms of struggle

Using the list above, or additional patterns you've noticed in yourself, what are some of the thoughts you have, feelings you experience, or behaviours you demonstrate, that indicate you may be struggling?

My Example

Neglecting my physical appearance and allowing myself to go multiple days in a row without showering

A persistent desire to be alone, feeling like I have no energy or patience to socialize, and being full of excuses to avoid my commitments like my weekly men's team meeting, scheduled phone calls, or social gatherings (especially if I think or know that they will ask me uncomfortable questions about my situation)

Burying myself in work projects and not enjoying it

Substance abuse and addiction (for me, this reveals itself when I can't control when, or in what context, I get high. For example, even though my men's team has a standard of being sober during sessions, when I'm in the basement, I will have no problem getting high before the meeting and not telling anyone about it)

YOUR TURN

Q: What are some of the indicators in my life that I'm struggling?

Feel free to go into as much detail as needed. I've been paying attention to these patterns in myself for the last ten years, so if it helps to make a note on your phone, and or open a page in your journal to vomit whatever comes to mind, I highly recommend it. From there, you can pinpoint the few patterns of behaviour that are most common and that you can use for your "If this, then that "action plan. ☯[25]

2.2 "If this, then that" action plan to struggle

---

25 ☯ **Philosophy Footnote:** *"Don't use your head as a filing cabinet."* **- Jim Rohn**

My example

1. Send a "I think I'm struggling" text to my buddy on my men's team and our team's group chat (example below)
2. Send Mohsin an e-transfer of $500 and have him send it back to me only when I've successfully gone a minimum of 14 days free of whatever addiction or substance is in control of me versus me being in control of it (mine tends to be weed, but it could be tobacco, sugar, alcohol, sex, porn, video games, Netflix, etc.)
3. Book an hour appointment to be completed within seven days with my counsellor

"I think I'm struggling," text example:

"I don't want you to worry and there's nothing I need right from you at this moment, but I'm not feeling like myself lately. I think I'm struggling with my mental health and want you to be aware. Would you be open to jumping on a call to talk in the next 24-48 hours?"

The purpose of this message is not to burden anyone in your life or have them try to solve your problems. A message like this is useful because it bridges the gap between you tackling your struggles alone and knowing that you have someone in your court you can lean on.

Key Point: Engage your men immediately. Do not tackle struggles alone.

Attacking a mental health struggle alone is like playing team deathmatch in Call of Duty 10 v 1. Technically, you could win. But you're more likely to be shot within 10 seconds of spawning. If you go ahead with this alone, it's you against addiction, masks, doubt, anxiety, stress, and the momentum of whatever direction you're headed. Once the other team gets a few kills under their belt, all of a sudden they have UAV, airstrikes, dogs, and you're in deep fucking shit.

Another way to think of struggling is like taking steps up or down a ladder. Every time doubt, fear, and addiction win, you're taking one step up a rung. The higher you allow yourself to climb, the harder it is to climb down, or, the more painful it is when you fall off. Think of engaging the men in your life and choosing to be helped, like taking a step down a rung. The sooner you allow yourself the gift of being helped and your men the gift of helping, the quicker you step off the ladder completely, and ultimately thrive with your mental health.

Your Turn

Q: When I notice that I am struggling I can and I will:

1.
2.
3.

Key Point: The more uncomfortable and difficult the decision, the closer you're moving towards recovery and control.

When you're struggling with your mental health, the easiest decisions tend to also be the most destructive. When you're in the basement, it's easier to reach for the joint or the liquor than it is to honour the truth that you're addicted. It's easier to choose skipping your team meeting than it is to choose showing up and talking about your struggle. And it's easier to put your mask on for protection than it is to take it off with your men.

It's in these moments where the uncomfortable decisions lead you back to the path of your thriving mental health. For me, I know that the more control I give weed, the worse the high feels and the worse I feel about myself. And that my default behaviour is to want to be alone and not have to confront the reality of my situation.

These behaviours in response to struggle only serve to make it more and more challenging to regain control over my mindset and my daily actions. Choose the uncomfortable path and choose to engage the men in your life you trust to show up for you when you need it most.

Once we understand that everyone has mental health, it becomes immediately clear that not asking for help from the people who care about you, as well as from professionals trained to be a pillar of strength in these moments, would be like breaking your arm and never going to the doctor for a cast.

Additionally, it's important to note that, while a men's team or the men you trust are an excellent support tool, they're not mental health professionals. Therefore, although we can rely on these men *absolutely*, we can't rely on them *exclusively*. Depending on your signs and symptoms, as well as how far you've allowed yourself to climb up the ladder of struggle, engaging with mental health professionals as soon as possible may be necessary.

With so many options, who to call can easily be overwhelming. My suggestion is to start with whichever resource is most accessible. That could be your family doctor, a help line, or an online counselling service like betterhelp.com. Other options include:

Psychiatrists
Psychologists
Psychiatric nurse practitioners
Physician assistants
Registered nurses
Social workers and more

Once you've taken the first step to engage a professional, you can explore different options from there. The most important thing to remember is to act on getting help now.

If, at first, you don't find a men's team you resonate with, or a mental health professional that makes you feel comfortable, change it. This is your life. There is no problem too small to bring to a professional. If you injured your shoulder you could get acupuncture, physiotherapy, try a chiropractor or hire a personal trainer. There's no right answer. Start with whatever is most accessible and you're most comfortable with, and, if the first resource you try isn't effective, don't give up. Try another.

You deserve to thrive and all men will benefit from you accessing help and making forward progress with your mental health. ☯[26]

Crisis

I experienced a real life emergency back in 2015. I was at a local Home Depot picking up flowers for our family's garden wearing flip flops, a tank top, and my old blue Town of Bradford lifeguard hat. At the checkout counter, I struck up a conversation with a woman named Julie. She suddenly gasped, grabbed her chest, and fell to the floor. I'd never experienced an emergency in all my years of being a lifeguard until this moment.

Remembering my training, I knelt beside her and found out she had just had a pacemaker installed. She felt massive pain and pressure in her chest and shoulder, and I thought she may be having a heart attack. I turned to the employee behind the counter and said, "You in the orange shirt, we need the ambulance on the phone. Use your radio to get a first aid kit and defibrillator immediately. "Next, I commanded the man to my left, "You with the glasses, I need you to keep everyone out of this area until the ambulance comes. "And finally, I turned back to Julie to reassure her that I was here for her and that everything was going to be okay.

Julie, I later found out, had a heart attack that day. She lived and soon recovered. While it was scary in the moment, that experience taught me a valuable lesson in what a physical health crisis looks like and how to deal with it. In an emergency, community resources are useful, but they're not enough. More importantly, look at what happened to Julia during the crisis; she fell to the floor gasping for air and was virtually *helpless*.

The definition of a mental health crisis is that there is an immediate risk of harming myself or someone else. Therefore, we need to remember that in a crisis, you, or whoever is experiencing the crisis,

---

26 ☯ **Philosophy Footnote:** *"Tend to the part of the garden that you can reach."* **- Jack Kornfield**

is not in control. This is an emergency situation. In my experience, it would have been negligent of me to say, "Don't worry, I'm a lifeguard! I'll handle this. "Or worse, to think that Julie would handle it on her own while on the floor unable to breathe. Crisis situations are why we have police, ambulance, and fire departments. They almost never happen, and because of that it's easy to let your guard down or to not take it seriously.

In 2019, my dad got a call from the wife of one of his best friends who said that her husband didn't seem like himself that morning. She said he was talking to himself, had mentioned suicide, and didn't know where he was. They immediately called the police and my dad jumped in his car and drove towards their house. When my dad found him, he was walking directly along a set of train tracks. If his wife hadn't called my dad and the police immediately, he may have died that day. Mental health crises do not mean you or the other person is crazy, it means you're out of control. Calling emergency services immediately is the most important action we can take in these moments.

3.1 Signs and symptoms of crisis

Examples of signs and symptoms that you or someone in your life is experiencing a crisis include, but are not limited to:

- **Sleeplessness**
- **Ritualistic preoccupation with certain activities**
- **Increased suspiciousness and paranoia**
- **Unpredictable outbursts**
- **Increased hostility**
- **Verbal threats**
- **Angry staring or grimacing.**
- **Suicidal ideation, both thoughts as well as planning**

I've never personally been in a crisis with my mental health and because the definition of a crisis is that you're out of control, there's no way to know for sure what you will feel or do if that situation ever arises. Therefore, it's best to simply remind ourselves that it's a possibility and to defer to experts' opinions.

3.2 "If this, then that" action plan for crisis

Please consider following these guidelines outlined by the mental health charity Jack.org. If you know someone who is in immediate danger of harming themselves or others as a result of a mental health crisis, call 9-1-1 and/or follow this plan if you're not certain:

Step 1: Identify the risk of harm by asking yourself or the other person direct questions

- **Are you thinking of suicide or hurting yourself?**
- **Do you have a plan or have you been researching one?**

Do not be concerned about giving someone ideas they may not have had. If they have been thinking about suicide or self-harm, it's imperative that you, and emergency services, know this. Direct questions like these will allow you to decide quickly the severity of the situation so that you can either call 9-1-1 or take the following steps below.

Step 2: If possible, stay with them and get another trusted adult involved

- **Remove any objects that could be harmful that are within reach.**
- **Engage your mental health supports or ask if they have a therapist, social worker, or counsellor they typically speak with so that you can help them get connected.**
- **Reach out to another trusted adult or a crisis line, and, if you're supporting someone, make sure that you have the support you need and are not putting yourself in harm's way by being there.**

A mental health support who knows this person's history can bring a lot more insight regarding what may be helpful for them in a crisis. If they do not have someone they work with and there is no immediate threat to their health or your own, getting a crisis line or someone with mental health expertise will be dramatically helpful.

Try these options or quickly research mental health crisis lines in your area:

1. Toronto and GTA: Google "Mental health crisis line" and CAMH Crisis Resources should be one of your first options for the GTA - https://www.camh.ca/en/health-info/crisis-resources
2. Canada Wide: Google "Mental health crisis lines Canada" for national resources on the canada.ca website - https://www.canada.ca/en/public-health/services/mental-health-services/mental-health-get-help.html
3. International Options: Google "International mental health crisis lines" for options in many countries around the world or type this link https://checkpointorg.com/global/
4. Curated List: Wikipedia has a large curated list of crisis lines by researching "list of suicide crisis lines wikipedia" or typing https://en.wikipedia.org/wiki/List_of_suicide_crisis_line

Step 3: If you think you or the person might be in immediate danger of harming themselves, you can

- Walk into, or walk them into, an emergency room to connect them to medical help
- Call 9-1-1 and ask if there is a mobile crisis unit in your area
- Recognizing that the police may not always feel like the safest option for some communities, connect with a local mental health support if possible

Everyone and anyone has the capacity to experience a crisis, and, in these cases, it is always appropriate to be safe rather than sorry. You or a friend may experience positive or thriving mental health for virtually all of your life and yet still have the capacity to be in crisis. Do not sweep it under the rug. Ensure you take the appropriate actions outlined above and keep your personal health and safety the highest priority.

Here's an abbreviated version of the tips above:

Mental Health Crisis Action Plan

1. **Be calm and direct.**
2. **Ask questions like, "Have you thought about suicide or harming yourself?" or "Do you have a plan or have been researching one?" to gauge the severity of the situation.**
3. **If possible, stay with them and get a mental health professional, or trusted adult involved immediately.**
4. **Walk yourself or them into an emergency room for medical help, call 9-1-1, or a crisis unit in your area.**
5. **Be safe rather than sorry, for yourself and for those experiencing a crisis.**

THE THREE STEPS TO SUCCESS

One of the most influential mentors in my life told me that success is actually very easy. He said there's only three steps:

1. **Choose a battlefield**
2. **Create a battleplan**
3. **Execute the plan**

In this context, success is defined as your thriving mental health and whatever that looks like for you. And if you have followed along up to this point (I encourage you to go back and complete the exercises if you haven't), you now have a practical and actionable plan for addressing your unique signs and symptoms to stress, struggle and even a crisis.

The "If this, then that "prompts, paired with your new awareness, means that you have a strategy for managing, experimenting with, and improving your responses to the dynamic changes in your mental health throughout your life.

Everyone's life situation is different and you will inevitably experience moments in your life that come with more intense experiences of stress. You may be a student going through a grewling semester. You may be a brand new father and haven't slept properly for months. Or you may have just lost a loved one and are grieving intensely. No matter the experience, in the context of men's mental health and masculinity, the same wind blows on us all. The difference in where your life turns out has much less to do with what happens as it does with what we do about it.

This is your opportunity to consciously choose your response. When life throws you a curve ball or you're on the court with a skilled opposing team, what plays will you call? Will you choose to make votes in the direction of your new life, engage men you trust in supporting you, and ask for help? Or will you choose your old ways of being and acting based on the wiring that all you need to do is man up? You now have the plan, so the choice is yours.

MY BATTLE PLAN

This one-pager is your cheat sheet to your thriving mental health. You can simply fill in the blanks below or you can write it out on your phone as I have. I have completed the example first and the next page is your opportunity to fill in.

Instructions:

1. **Fill in the mantra or the statement you designed in chapter three in order to anchor you to who you need to be, or how you need to think, in order to call into existence your new life.**
2. **Move your new "If this, then that" statements into the blanks provided below.**
3. **Close with a quote that inspires you to be your best self.**

My Thriving Mental Health Example

I am grateful for my relaxed, strong, and playful mind, body and spirit.

When I notice I am stressed, I can and I will:

1. **Lay down on the floor and breath deeply for 5-10 minutes relaxing my mind and body**
2. **Go for a walk outside and listen to my favourite relaxing music or call someone I love**
3. **Write down three things I'm grateful for and send an appreciation text or video to a friend**

If I notice I am struggling, I can and I will:

1. **Send a "I think I'm struggling" text to my buddy on my men's team and our team's group chat within 24 hours**
2. **Send Mohsin an e-transfer of $500 and have him send it back to me only when I've successfully gone a minimum of 14 days free of from my addiction**
3. **Book an hour appointment to be completed within seven days with my counsellor**

If I believe I'm losing control of my thoughts, feelings, or behaviours I can and I will:

1. **Call my mom, dad, or trusted adult immediately**
2. **Call 9-1-1 if necessary**

"You can have more than you've got because you can become more than you are." Jim Rohn

Your Thriving Mental Health

Mantra:

When I notice I am stressed, I can and I will:

1.
2.
3.

If I notice I am struggling, I can and I will:

1.
2.
3.

If I believe I'm losing control of my thoughts, feelings, or behaviours I can and I will:

1.
2.

Quote:

Key Point: Mental health and mental illness are not the same.

While everyone has mental health, not everyone has mental illness. Mental health is the state of your thoughts, feelings, and behaviours and mental illness is a cluster of symptoms that impact a person's mental wellbeing. An in-depth synopsis of each mental illness, like depression, obsessive compulsive disorder, bipolar disorder, and many others that can impact an individual's wellbeing, is outside the scope of this book. What is most important to remember is that, if you have identified a potential struggle in yours, or another's mental health, seek professional care as you would with any physical health distress.

Circle Up

In this first of four chapters designed to give you the practical tools needed in order to construct the Castle and life of your dreams, you learned the essentials of self-care. Alan Watts in his lecture series *Out of Your Mind* on Audible, points out that the Chinese character for 'man' is two sticks leaning against each other. It's this interconnectedness that can generate the desire for men to be generous, charitable, and invest in each other's success and wellbeing.

Furthermore, it simultaneously reveals the importance of learning to effectively take care of ourselves. If 'man' is fundamentally two sticks leaning against each other, and you're not a stick, but a floppy noodle, how can you be there to help another man? If you're in the basement and can't get off the couch, how can anyone else count on you? How can your family look to you to provide and protect? They can't. In the same series, he also stated, "If you want to spread delight, then you need to be more or less delightful. "

This "two sticks "visual from Alan Watts, combined with the following idea from Jim Rohn, makes up our philosophy of self-care here at Circle Up, "I will take care of me, so that I can take care of you, if you would please take care of you, so that you can take care of me. "

Think about your new battle plan for thriving mental this way; what does the flight attendant advise you to do during an emergency? ☯[27]

---

27 ☯ **Philosophy Footnote:** *"You are no use in helping others get their masks on until you have yours secured." - Iain Gabriel*

They instruct you to put on your oxygen mask first so that you can then help others around you. Or imagine you're a glass of water, how can you pour love, and light, and energy into the lives of your men and communities if you have an empty glass? You can't. Iain loves this analogy and always reminds me, "If you value filling up other people's cups, then you have a moral responsibility to make sure that yours runneth over. "

All of these perspectives, especially the dynamic nature of my mental health, have served me in establishing self-care practices that work for me. I offer them to you now in the hopes that you'll design your own mental health action plan.

Another major emphasis we explored on self-care was the responsibility to put yourself in a position to be taken care of. With our default context of "man up, "avoid, deflect, and protect yourself with your mask, this is the most difficult practice of changing the way we think, feel, and act on our mental health. Every word of this book was intentionally designed to help you normalize asking for help and being there for the men you care about. Now, in chapter five, we put this philosophy into practice.

Circle Up!

Medellin, Colombia - April 2021

CHAPTER SUMMARY

The Chinese character for 'man' is fundamentally two sticks leaning against each other. It's this interconnectedness that exposes the importance of learning to effectively take care of ourselves. If 'man' is two sticks leaning against each other, and you're not a stick, but a floppy noodle, how can you be there to help another man? No sports team would ever go into battle without a strategy, yet we run onto the battlefield of our lives every day without a plan for the inevitable adversites, struggles, and even crises we face. Prepare yourself to be strong in the face of life's challenges by developing your own unique mental health action plan. Taking care of yourself is your greatest contribution to the world.

RESOURCE SUMMARY

Stay close to the resources, quotes, and thinkers you resonated most with in this chapter. Pay attention to what speaks to your heart. If you said to yourself, "I should check that out, "take action immediately.

1. **Jack Talks - Instagram - @jack.org - Jack.org**
2. **"Learn This Skill Or Live A Mediocre Life" - YouTube - By Jim Rohn**
3. *Atomic Habits* **- By James Clear**
4. **Out of Your Mind -** Audible.com **- By Alan Watts**
5. **Instagram - @ericwindeler - Eric Windeler**

SELF-REFLECTION OPPORTUNITY

Once complete, move these notes to your phone. This will serve to summarize what you have learned, as well as ensure the resources, quotes, and ideas you personally resonated with most, are available at your fingertips.

Key points to remember (fill in here):

Who is someone that I trust to reach out to with an "I'm struggling" text if I feel that I'm struggling with my mental health?

What is one idea from this chapter that will help me "set a better sail" in my own personal philosophy?

CHAPTER FIVE:

MASCULINE CARE: A MENTAL HEALTH REVOLUTION

"Greater love has no one than this: to lay down one's life for one's friends."
John 15:13

GIVING A FUCK

"Jonathan, "Paul opened, "How old are you now? "

Congruent with most transformational seminars I had ever attended, the first day of Reborn was twelve hours so I replied lamely, sleep deprivation clearly present in my tone, "twenty-two, why? "

"Really... "I could see he was doing some mental math as he countered, "When's your birthday? "

Still unsure as to why he was asking, I responded, "Only a few months away. February 3rd, if you really want to know. "

Apparently, it was important information because he took out his phone and made a note. Paul was a friend of my parents and I'd met him before at business events in the past. He's a 6'5 tower of a man and so his body was too big for a single seat. His left leg had me almost falling out of my chair. We were meeting again for the first time in years while attending the personal development seminar *Reborn* hosted by a young Tony Robbins-esque entrepreneur named Armin Shaffe.

Armin, easily one of the most energizing, inspiring, and high-potential men I had ever met, changed my life that day. In a moment of destiny, his seminar had me in the same room as Paul, and I was reborn by the simplest of questions, “How old are you? ”

“I’m going to call you on your birthday, ”he said. “I think you’ll be happy I did. ”

I didn’t hear from Paul again for another three months. Then, as promised, on my birthday I got the call that became the gift I never knew I needed. He invited me to be his guest for something he called the *Men’s Weekend*. Apparently, you needed to be at least twenty-three years old to attend, and, while I was already reading books, attending Toastmasters every week, and volunteering with Jack.org, I didn’t take for granted the integrity necessary to write down my birthday and actually follow up with me when I turned twenty-three.

Paul gave-a-fuck enough to think about me and call. So, I went. And my life has never been the same since. The course was meeting bi-weekly for eight sessions and I was invited to attend as a guest for three of their meetings. On my first night, they asked me to bring a prop representing something I was proud of. I brought the goal post I had made with my girlfriend at the time, on New Years of 2018, which represented my visions for my future.

That group, which was the first men’s circle I had ever attended, gave me the opportunity to share why it was important to me. I talked about how, in High School, I felt lost and hopeless, how I had no direction, and how my family and Jim Rohn helped me find the strength to believe in myself and start dreaming again.The experience was both re-affirming that I was on the right path and tremendously uplifting to see other men share their pride and a part of their lives with the circle. I had never seen a group of men come together and be so vulnerable.

That night, we laughed, we cried, and I said “fuck it ”and accepted their invitation to do the Men’s Weekend that was to happen a few months later. Another investment in myself, it turned out, became another one of the best decisions of my life. Years later, with these words pouring out of me about men's mental health and masculinity, I can't help but think of a line from *Shantaram* when one of the main characters, Karla, said, "If fate doesn't make you laugh, then you just don't get the joke. "

Sitting here now, remembering my decision to have faith and say "fuck it, "I smile and laugh with gratitude at fate and its mysterious ways. In *The Alchemist*, Paulo Coelho wrote, "When someone makes a decision, he is really diving into a strong current that will carry him to places he had never dreamed of when he first made the decision. "

In the following pages, we'll discuss:

1. **How as men, we're stronger together**
2. **How to take your mask off safely and**
3. **How to provide masculine care and giving a fuck about another man**

In the three years that followed that first guest night with Paul and the Men's Weekend, I learned the second of three major pillars in constructing a life you love: finding the men who've got your back no matter what.

Building masculine relationships is a mental health revolution. It's been said that if you want to go fast, go alone. But if you want to go far, go together. This chapter is about doing the challenging and uncomfortable work of developing and investing in the masculine relationships that will take your life further than you could have ever imagined.

STRONGER TOGETHER

Sometimes, self-care isn't enough. Sometimes, you take massive arrows and the only thing that can help you heal from your wounds is being held by the people you love. And sometimes, it takes seeing the men around you doing well to fuel the fire of your own beliefs. I've been experimenting with accountability long before I ever heard of a men's team and it's taught me that we're stronger together.

The Gestalt Principle

Most of this chapter emphasizes the direct mental health benefits of masculine relationships, like having a space to take off your mask, so I will start with the indirect. Iain has been beating into me for the last couple years the idea of the Gestalt principle. This field of psychology argues that the whole is greater than the sum of its parts. In other words, instead of 1 + 1 = 2, 1 + 1 = 3 or even greater. Therefore, increasing the number of parts, or brothers, actually amplifies the sum of the output and experience, rather than simply adding to it. When you have strong men around you who are competent and successful, it feeds into your success, health and happiness. ☯[28]

From this perspective, every time your life gets better and you become more successful, the lives of the men around you do too. In the exact same way, as the men in your life do better, so will you. This is an excellent argument for developing masculine relationships, because, not only will you have more fun in your life, but by investing in the men around you, you will also have more success. Counter intuitive to the "men are always in the competition "belief system we grew up with, Iain likes to describe Gestalt and this philosophy as baking the biggest pie possible.

Instead of looking to get the biggest slice of the pie you can, focus on helping the men around you be successful, thereby creating a bigger pie for everyone. Our collective success, as the Gestalt framework suggests, is a much greater pie overall than the sum of its parts could ever be. I find this pie analogy useful any time I find myself living in fear, scarcity, or jealousy towards other men. Again, with Iain being my best friend and having so much potential, I often find myself self-conscious and looking for scraps of pie falling off the table. I know this way of thinking and being is not only destructive to our friendship, but, selfishly, not in my best interest. ☯[29]

---

28 ☯ **Philosophy Footnote:** *"Shift your mindset from scarcity to one of abundance. A smaller slice of the new pie you create with the people in your life can be exponentially larger than a bigger slice of the current one."* **- Iain Gabriel**

29 ☯ **Philosophy Footnote:** *"This is something that Jonathan and I have discussed at length. The fact that you are reading my words in Jonathan's book is testament to him having applied this shift in philosophy in his life."* **- Iain Gabriel**

Referring back to the warrior's allegory from chapter one, the warrior knows it's in his best interest to have the men around him prepared, strong and healthy. In this analogy, I'm not worried nearly as much about how much pie I'm getting as keeping my limbs on the battlefield. The warrior always wants the strongest, most competent men at his side, and, so should you.

Not only will you get more pie, because the Gestalt principle will create more for everyone, but you'll keep your arms. When we can shift our focus to gratitude for having amazing men in our lives, we can stop agonizing about who's in competition with who and start opening doors of opportunity and investing in our people.

THE SUCKHOLE

In my experiences with both Landmark and the Men's Weekend, they introduced a concept that relates to the basement called the World Sucks Chart. This illustration shows that the closer you are to the suckhole (the whole in the bottom), meaning the more you're focused on yourself as an individual, the closer you are to doubt, feeling like a victim, and like your problems are insurmountable.

This concept of the suckhole has two major benefits and is one of the reasons why being on a men's team is so valuable. First, when you focus on helping a cause greater than yourself, like in a relationship with one of your men, or even higher on the chart, like with your team, it forces you to expand your thinking and your skill sets. When you focus on solving the challenges your team faces, your individual challenges become much less important.

Think about how this relates to your purpose. If your purpose is to get out of bed in the morning, how inspired do you think you'll be to get on the battlefield in your life? But if you're on a team with men, and your purpose as a group is to make a difference in your community, think about how that simple change in perspective will impact your attitude, energy, and focus.

The point of intentionally choosing to move yourself higher on the World Sucks chart is that your energy flows where you focus your attention. This became crystal clear to me when I started advocating for youth mental health. By focusing on a cause greater than myself, my character was molded by the needs of the community rather than just out of meeting my basic needs. Instead of setting my focus on making enough money to pay my rent, I was developing leadership and communication skills that make me highly valuable, while making a difference in the world. This adjustment in your focus can become a major asset in improving your mental health. Author, legendary sales trainer, and speaker, Zig Ziglar, used to always say that, "if you help enough other people pay their bills, all of yours will be taken care of. "☯[30]

The second practical aspect of choosing to move up in the World Sucks chart, by focusing on taking care of your community, your team, or someone you care about, is that you will find yourself surrounded by people who can take care of you. This give and take is the major theme of finding your men. Not only will you become a better man by focusing on community, but when you're personally getting too close to the suckhole or the basement, your men will be there to help pull you out.

The basement is where you can't get off the couch, you're living in your head, and the voice of addiction becomes the loudest. If you get too close, the monkeys begin to convince you why it's okay to quit drinking tomorrow instead of today and help you rationalize that your current behaviour isn't all that bad. In our men's circle, we call this bullshitting ourselves. It's why we have a men's team to begin with. These men know you better than anyone else. So when you're in the basement, full of monkeys, doubt and addiction, and when reaching out for help is the most challenging, you've already put yourself in a position to be cared for.

---

30 ☯ **Philosophy Footnote:** *"If you focus on helping the people in your life and community fill their cups, yours will be filled by default."* **- Iain Gabriel**

These men have your best interest in mind and will be able to hold up a mirror helping to reveal the damage you're causing yourself and others by consistently buying your own bullshit. I like to think of this benefit as being like a stop-loss order in investing stocks. Instead of letting your stocks drop below a certain price, the stop-loss automatically sells your investment for you so you don't lose all your money. Having men around you who you trust to call you out on your bullshit, is like having a stop-loss for struggling on the mental health spectrum. Before you ever fall too deep into the basement, these men can help you shift your focus back to your purpose, what you're committed to, and the difference you can make in the world by choosing intentionally where you want to focus on the World Sucks chart.

For The Boys

Your men are more than a resource for asking for help. These men, when invested in and cared for, will help add colour, shenanigans, and ultimately remind you that life isn't all that serious. If it wasn't for the broskis, I'd never have gone to my first music festival. If it wasn't for my homies, I'd probably still be the kid with no social life, calling himself the "5 a.m. hustle, "and going to bed at 8 p.m. every night. This work is about the men. But it's also about the boys, you know? ☯[31]

How To Take Off Your Mask Safely

In chapter three, we answered the "what "in the question "What do we need to do to serve men who're struggling with mental health? " That answer was derived from the understanding that, as men, we believe the notion that because our struggle makes us weak and less of a man, we need to wear masks to protect ourselves and the world from our truth. As a result, this entire book has been challenging you to consciously recondition the way you think about your mental health from man up to Circle Up.

---

31 ☯ **Philosophy Footnote:** *"Greater love has no one than this: to lay down one's life for one's friends."* **- John 15:13**

The only problem left now is that with the rest of the world still thinking and sowing the seeds of struggle equals weakness, you're left with the task of consciously seeking, and/or creating, the environments and relationships that are conducive to you safely taking off your mask. If you can do that, you will have the freedom to be honest with yourself and your men. Rather than struggle alone, and face the ball and shackle of the basement without help, you will be empowered to reach out to pillars of strength in times of challenge. The men in your life can become your secret weapon, like wind feeding your sails, taking you further than ever before.

Let's think of the foundation needed in order to establish an effective mask-down environment with the same context encouraged by Michael Pollan in his book on psychedelics, *How To Change Your Mind: What The New Science of Psychedelics Teaches Us About Consciousness, Dying, Addiction, Depression, and Transcendence.* His research surfaces that, in order to have the best chance at an empowering trip, it's critical to intentionally curate your set and setting— set, referring to one's mindset going into the experience, and setting, referring to the physical and social environment in which one chooses to trip.

The exact same thinking can be applied to masculine relationships and creating the conditions for taking off your mask. First, unlike a friendship, where most of the shared experiences are fun and casual, cultivating mask-down environments that you can count on for truth seeking, are, first and foremost, about having uncomfortable conversations. It's not that you can't do this with friends. You can. But with these relationships in particular, the mindset and context going in is that the entire purpose is to be able to face your addictions, look at your arrows, and take off your mask.

This is the reason why friendships can often be strained when someone is struggling with their mental health. One friend feels that they are burdening the other, or the supporting friend feels burdened like there is too much give and not enough take. That common barrier to dropping masks does not exist with masculine relationships because you've established up front the purpose of the space, and this relationship, is to have these conversations. How brilliant.

Therefore, while I am not advocating that you lie to friends about how you feel, I am encouraging you to follow the principles outlined in this chapter to establish a few relationships dedicated to the ongoing betterment of your mental, physical, and spiritual health. These men become a sort of mastermind for your mutual success where anything is on table and the expectation every time you connect is that it will be a safe space to be vulnerable and honest.

Next, think of setting as the nuance to know the time and place to take off your mask. In a psychedelic trip, you want to control as many variables as possible to eliminate fear, stress, or interruption. For example, my best trips have been with friends I trust in a calming and controlled setting, like inside, or in a secluded spot in nature. The last place you'd want to trip, and I know this from personal experience (no idea what we were thinking), is while riding a bicycle on a bridge with cars driving fast and loudly beside you at 100km/h.

This is mostly just good common sense. The last place the warrior would want to remove his mask is in the middle of the battlefield. So, for you, looking to effectively design an environment for taking off your mask, start by being thoughtful about your set and setting. I like to start, whenever possible, with 100% privacy. That means only men you know and trust are part of the conversation.

Then, consider how you can play with your environment to induce feelings of intimacy, introspection, and vulnerability. Some of the most important mask-down conversations I've had in my life were in the darkness of night circling up around a fire. The fire provides the perfect visual distraction to reduce any defensiveness that arises from direct eye-contact, as well symbolically represents rebirth and transformation. For thousands of years, men have been meeting around fires to talk about their struggles and arrows. I encourage you to tap into that ancestral wisdom and see how being intentional about your setting impacts your ability to honour the truth.

Honouring the Truth

The key to being able to take your mask off is to remember why you're doing any of this. What's your intention? What's the context for wanting to take your mask off in the first place? How will it serve you and, therefore, serve everyone else in your life? If you can remember that as men, we're least likely to ask for help when we need it most, and make a commitment to choose a different direction, you will find the men and the spaces where you can honour the truth in the face of struggle.

In the context of men's mental health, I've found that the most important commitment we can make is to be honest with ourselves about where we're at and how we're doing. Generally speaking, in the men's work, we discuss five-pillars to a masculine relationships:

1. **Trust**
2. **Confidentiality**
3. **Respect**
4. **Commitment**
5. **Fun**

The ultimate goal is to find men you trust *completely*. Trust dissolves all barriers to honesty because you know, without a shadow of a doubt, this man has your best interest in mind. All of my biggest breakthroughs, like the experience with my dad in the introduction, as well as with Iain in chapter three, have been when I've been able to drop my mask completely. Trusting another man helps you transcend any anxiety about judgement, fear that what you say may be repeated outside of the relationship, and most importantly, break through the conditioned beliefs that your struggle makes you weak.

For starters, trust, which is our highest priority, is not possible without confidentiality. You can probably think of a time when you told someone something in confidence and that trust was broken. How did it make you feel? It likely made you question the dependability of the relationship and what else you've shared that was eventually repeated. From that point forward, you start to wear your mask a little tighter, filtering what you do and what you say to avoid the embarrassment or pain associated with distrust.

You lose all of the benefits of masculine relationships and a men's team without confidentiality. When there's no confidentiality, and as a result, no trust, a man shows up with his ego, wearing a mask, and doesn't reveal the roots of what's bothering him or holding him back in his life. He tends to want to look good and, therefore, doesn't share where he's out of honour with his integrity or where the grips of addiction have a tight hold on him. This is a tragedy. Honouring the truth is necessary to bridge the gap between the man you are today and the man you've always wanted to be.

If you wear your mask in these spaces, your presence becomes a waste of time for you as well as for all the men involved. When we avoid the full truth for fear of looking bad, all the advice or solutions we generate about what to do in our lives have little value. Half truths, in the context of generating ideas for your better future, can only create solutions incongruent with your reality. If you don't meet yourself where you're at, how could you take yourself where you want to go?

On Episode #50 of my Circle Up podcast, Iain linked wearing your mask in this context to trying to bake a pie, but lying to yourself about what ingredients are available (not sure his obsession with pies are). He said if you're seeking solutions for your addictions, arrows, and bad habits by listing a bunch of ingredients you don't actually have in your house, the men who care about you enough to listen will start offering suggestions and recipes that are virtually irrelevant. How could they help? You don't even have the ingredients!

To help you and your men in the process of developing trust for mask-down conversations, I'll offer you the same framework for confidentiality that was given to me. Since joining my first men's team, I've heard the phrase, "Everything you say, see, hear, and do in this space is confidential "hundreds of times. Today, knowing it's importance, I would never start a meeting without it.

Here's an example of standards of confidentiality you can use in your life:

1. **Everything you see, hear, say and do here is confidential.**
2. **Share the lessons; the names are confidential.**
3. **There are circles of confidentiality; what is said in one circle is confidential from another.**
4. **The only exception is in the service of the other man**

Number four is especially critical inside the context of mental health. As we've outlined previously, a mental health crisis is when someone is at imminent risk of injuring themselves or someone else. In this case, confidentiality must be breached for the safety of this person's environment. Some men criticize that this emphasis on confidentiality is overkill, but it's not.

The matters at hand during a one-on-one conversation or in an effective men's circle are not inconsequential. If you're visualizing you and your buddies sitting at a bar or shooting the shit over a beer, think again. We're not sitting around joking about the time you shit your pants at the Mandarin restaurant, we're coming together to have the conversations about what's holding you back from becoming a successful, healthy, and self-sufficient man for yourself and your family. It's not that there's no place for fun, there is. It's just secondary to the primary purpose of becoming the man you've always wanted to be.

These masculine relationships are about where we are struggling and the negative impact it's having on our lives. Men often express that they were able to share information about themselves they've never felt comfortable sharing. That is only because of the confidentiality maintained in these circles. Without it, a man cannot, and I want to stress, should not, take off their mask in front of those men.

Key Point: Learn to tip your mask.

As Brene Brown said, "When you trust someone, you're choosing to risk making something you value (in our case, your arrows, addictions, and vulnerabilities) vulnerable to another person's actions." Therefore, in the same way that you wouldn't ask a stranger to hold your briefcase full of a million dollars while you took a shit, you shouldn't give a man more trust than he's proven he can handle.

This is where learning to tip your mask, versus removing it completely, is a great strategy in the process of finding men you trust with anything and everything. Billionaire Warren Buffet is known for saying, "Don't trust the depths of the river with both feet. "Learning to tip your mask over time is analogous to dipping one toe in the river, then a second toe, and finally the foot, before trusting the relationship to fully remove your mask in a space of ruthless compassion.

I remember a group meeting with almost a hundred men, when one man shared from the front of the room an incredibly vulnerable story about being sexually abused. Later, when we had the opportunity to connect one on one, he described his experience to me as feeling judged and even ridiculed by some of the other men. Does this mean men's circle's aren't giving men the benefit they desire? Possibly. But what I believe to be more likely is an error in judgement.

This man chose to tell an extremely vulnerable story in front of a room of strangers. Talk about risky. I definitely felt ashamed that the group didn't do a better job of holding space and honouring his vulnerability, but it became a valuable lesson for both him, and I, about learning to tip our masks over time with men rather than taking them off completely the first time we meet a group of strangers.

In another circle I participated in, the facilitator, Steve Richmond, who's a respected mentor of hundreds of men in our community said, "For the next eight weeks, take the risk of making the men in this room your men. "I believe he was spot on. Trusting another man is always a risk, therefore, it's important we take the process of choosing the men we will trust to have our backs no matter what, seriously.

Key Point: You attract what you are, not what you want.

Have faith that, if you give trust, you will get trust. And that, if you become a trustworthy person, you will attract trustworthy people into your life. I want to make it clear that I don't think you shouldn't trust men. My intention with this emphasis on trust is not to create further paranoia. It's simply to offer the path of least resistance to help seeking behaviours by developing a few key relationships where there's complete trust.

I believe that in the same way Jim Rohn said, "Success is not something you pursue, success is something you attract by the person you become. "You will only be able to attract trustworthy men by first becoming a trustworthy person. Therefore, if you intend to attract men into your life who are honest, who can maintain confidentiality, and will always have your best interest at heart, you will fare best by becoming the type of person who honours those values yourself. At this point in my life, I have more than a dozen men who I can call if I'm struggling. You too can have faith that as you practice this philosophy, and become the type of person who honours the truth, you will become a magnet to men seeking the same opportunity.

Providing Masculine Care

Over the past few years of my advocacy journey, many people have reached out to me asking, "How do I be there for someone in my life that's struggling? " Oftentimes, it's a man who is concerned about a friend, and, other times, it's a parent noticing changes in behaviour in their child. Regardless, the first resource I point people to is bethere.org.

Be There

Created by the team at Jack.org, Be There is the most engaging and comprehensive resource available to learn about how to support someone struggling with their mental health. As always, Jack.org is doing a phenomenal job of normalizing mental health conversations and offering practical tools you can implement in your life. Intuitively, both my dad when he supported me in high school, as well as Iain when he was there for me when I struggled with Noah's death, were using the Be There "golden rules."

The framework started when my good friend, Jesse Lee Haymen, who was also the Vice President of Jack.org at the time, and the Jack team, set out to create an experiential website where people of all backgrounds could come and hear stories from those who've had experience supporting a loved one struggling with their mental health. Since its launch, the website and framework have made a phenomenal impact and won multiple awards for its efforts in the global mental health landscape. When I'm in doubt about how to care for a man, or anyone in my life who's struggling, I first turn to Be There.

The five golden rules are:

1. **Say what you see**
2. **Show you care**
3. **Hear them out**
4. **Know your role**
5. **Connect to help**

They do an incredible job at making the rules simple on the website and so I highly recommend you bookmark bethere.org on your computer. That way, you can refer to it whenever you need. Additionally, we will explore a couple of the stories outlined in this book to offer more colour to the list above.

1. Say what you see

Saying what you see rather than your interpretation of what you see, is the first step to effective care. Iain didn't say to me, "Hey, man, you haven't been yourself lately and I think that means that you're struggling and depressed because of Noah's death." Instead he said, "Hey man, you haven't been yourself lately. I want you to know that I'm here for you, so let's listen to some music and hangout in the park." Notice the difference?

The first example makes a man guarded. The second makes a man feel welcomed. If a man in your life hasn't consciously shifted his context about his mental health, without even realizing what he's doing, he will raise his mask to protect his ego. In Iain's approach, he created the space for open dialogue without putting pressure on me to have a conversation I wasn't ready for.

Saying what you see is about the facts, not about your interpretation of what's happening. Approaching masculine care with assumptions or your interpretation, raises a man's guard. Pointing out what you've been noticing, shows you've been paying attention.

2. Show you care

The easiest way to show that you care is to tell someone. That could look like, "Hey, I noticed you've been (behaviour you're concerned about) and want you to know I care about you and am here for you if and whenever you need to talk. "The second, and more difficult way to show you care, is to actually give a fuck. To show up like my dad did, day after day.

It was my dad's actions, more than his words, that demonstrated that he was there for me. It was his desire for me to be at my best that inspired me to want more for my life again. Showing you care is as simple as showing up. If you truly want those you care about to thrive (which you should because when your environment improves, your life improves), it's often not enough to tell them; you need to show them.

Masculine care is about commitment. Like the warrior going to battle, you want the men you're going to war with to be at their best. Otherwise, they won't be able to hold their shield in line and take care of your back when *you* need it. With both Iain and my dad, they knew me well enough to know I wasn't at my best, then gave a fuck enough to invest in me and make sure that I was okay. In most cases, being there with each other is enough to show that you care, and really giving a fuck about another man shows up in your actions, not your words.

3. Hear them out

In chapter one, we explored monkeys and how when a microphone gets too close to a speaker it begins to resonate violently. That is where hearing a man out makes a world of a difference. Giving a man the space to share what's bothering him, and what arrows he's dealing with, quiets the monkeys and helps him put what he's experiencing into perspective. It's when we keep our arrows hidden from the world that the chattering monkeys get louder and louder.

In my experience, hearing a man out isn't necessarily about the words exchanged and more about the space created. Words can be useful when you're sorting through problems and looking for solutions, but when we lost Noah, there was no solution to be found. I wasn't dealing with a failing business or aching body, I was struggling with a massive arrow. I lost my nephew. When a man takes an arrow like that, hearing them out often looks like giving them the space to cry, scream, or express themselves in any way that's helpful. That's exactly what Iain did.

4. Know your role

Knowing your role means two things; first, that you're not an expert (unless you're a psychologist or psychotherapist, in which case, great, do your job), and second, not to act like one. Being there is about simply that, being there. It's not about giving advice or about solving a man's problems, it's about caring enough to take the uncomfortable step of saying what you see, showing you care, and hearing them out.

As soon as you step into the realm of giving a man advice, you're getting in the way of allowing them to feel the emotion behind their arrows. While it's appropriate to ask questions and be an active listener, more often than not, dispensing advice to a man who's not asking for it isn't helpful. The caveat being, like I said, if you're an expert in the area of their struggle or have direct lived experience where advice could help them avoid a major future misstep.

Knowing your role can also mean that you may not be the best person to help the man. You may initiate the conversation, show them you care, and find out that they're not comfortable talking to you about their arrows. That's perfectly okay and happens all the time. If this happens, what's important is that the man knows you care and that they're supported. Maybe another man is the right person for them to talk to. Maybe they just need time on their own.

Either way, our goal is to pattern interrupt the inherited context around men's mental health and masculinity by initiating conversations. It's almost guaranteed that it won't be perfect the first time and so don't give up on a man if they're wearing a mask and hiding from the root of their pain. It's part of the process of rewiring our thinking and is inevitable inside of our ongoing commitment to being there for each other.

5. **Connect to help**

If you or a man in your life are demonstrating signs and symptoms of a mental health struggle or crisis (refer to chapter four and the mental health spectrum), there's no action more important than connecting them to professional help. Your support, and the support of a community resource like a men's team, is most useful when we're stressed and dealing with the everyday challenges of our own lives. But we're not professionals.

From our new context that no man is alone and everyone has mental health and the capacity to struggle, there should be no shame in seeking help from a therapist, counselor, or other professional mental health resource. As discussed in chapter four, there's no stigma in calling an ambulance when you have a heart attack, so there should be no problems in speaking with a psychologist if you're struggling with mental health.

When seeking care or caring for another man, just like you would drive your friend to the hospital if he broke his leg and not try to put it back in place yourself, we want to be there for the men in our lives who are struggling, not fix them. This rule ties back into knowing your role. Cuts and scrapes and even small arrows can be healed together and on your men's teams, but spears or other significant injuries, like the loss of a child or a parent, can take a massive toll on a person's psyche and oftentimes require more comprehensive care.

Ruthless Compassion

The framework we use for masculine care in Circle Up is not only Be There, but also ruthless compassion. I offer both because you may resonate with one more than the other. This one in particular hits the nail on the head for men like me who're inspired by the warrior allegory we've explored in depth throughout this book. As a warrior, arrows go hand in hand with battle. They are an inevitability. No matter what decisions we make in life, or what battlefields we find ourselves on, we face trauma, pain, and tragedy.

I know men who've lost it all in their divorces. Their kids, their houses, their businesses, everything. My friends Nick, Iain, and Mike, lost their fathers to suicide. Others, like Eric Windeler and Bill Bagg, have lost their sons. My brother's son died tragically at birth. And I could go on and on. The point is that when men in your life take arrows, which they will, we have an opportunity to show up and take a stand for them.

Ruthless compassion isn't about solving a man's problems, for there's often nothing to solve. It's about making the commitment to ensure the men in your life are cared for. Imagine the warrior who came back from battle with a devastating injury and all of the men around him simply told him to walk it off and man up. He'd likely die in hours. In warrior culture, this would never happen. But it's what we do with our men.

In warrior culture, when you walked off the battlefield with injuries, men and their entire communities would come together to help you rest and heal. They would pick up any necessary slack in the short-term, until you found the strength to pick up your shield and fight again. Warriors would be honoured and respected. They're culture-recognized, as Alan Watts demonstrated with the Chinese symbol for 'man,' being essentially two sticks leaning on each other, the interdepence of every man in the tribe.

When the men in your life don't address their wounds, they weaken more and more through neglect. This impacts not only them directly, but their families, their communities, and you too. When you're on the battlefield and need a shield to your left, but the man hasn't healed from wounds in previous fights, you die. The death of a warrior's spirit doesn't occur in a silo. No man is an island.

Unfortunately, we seem to have become paralyzed by the decades of baggage associated with the "man up "motto that we've lost our common sense. And this concept actually transcends men because when anyone comes home injured from battle today, we pretend that the arrow doesn't hurt and that it isn't bleeding. And what do we do with these people? We let it slide. We can tell they're covering up their pain and expect them to brush it off, grab their sword and get back on the battlefield. We give them a few days off work and then ask if they'll be able to get us that report by Monday.

Where's the Compassion?

Compassion is when a community comes together and cooks to help a neighbour who's grieving the loss of a loved one. Or taking in a friend for six months because they lost their job and need a hand getting back on their feet. Compassion is being a good listener. Compassion is having empathy. Compassion is remembering that, as warriors, arrows are inevitable.

So, to have compassion as a warrior is to not only point out a man's bleeding arm, but to sit beside your brother and to tend to his wounds. It's not to shame the men around us for feeling the pain associated with the tragic loss of someone they love, but to hold them and reassure them that they're not alone in their grief. Finally, it's not to make our men feel inferior or weak for needing time to heal, but to remind them of the strength and courage it took for them to pick up their sword and shield in the first place and fight an honourable battle.

This is compassion, and it goes hand in hand with masculine care. This style of care builds bridges and brings men together. It's what I want to share with my friends and family when they're struggling. And what I hope to receive when I've fought bravely and taken arrows on the battlefield of my life. What I don't want, and what our warriors also don't need, is compassion alone. We need ruthless compassion.

Compassion isn't enough.

In my experience, compassion alone doesn't move the needle for men. It's like what Jim Rohn said about his early mentor Earl Shoaff: "If Earl wasn't blunt in those early days, I likely would have missed a lot of these lessons. "If you only deployed compassion with a warrior, he'd never recover his will to fight.

You'd hold him, feed him, and share positive words of affirmation. The only problem? He'd still have a fucking arrow lodged in his shoulder. At some point or another, in order to do what's best for the man, and in order for other men to do what's best for you, that arrow needs to be pulled. As warriors, we need to lead, and be led, back into action and onto the battlefield. Compassion alone breeds complacency. Ruthless compassion is the definition of masculine care.

Ruthlessness, when done correctly, doesn't force a man to hide out. It helps a man take off his mask. Standing eye to eye with one of your brothers in arms, communicating how much you care, and then pointing directly at the addictions and the arrows and asking him, "What are we going to do about this?" That's a masculine relationship. While it's important for us to have compassion for each other and give men the time and space to heal, it's just as important to have the difficult conversations where we address the struggles they're facing and the addictions they're bullshitting themselves about.

Compassion alone makes men soft. With compassion alone, we may never have the uncomfortable conversations a man needs to break through his struggle. But ruthlessness alone doesn't work either. Ruthlessness alone makes men defensive and engages their ego. Ruthlessness alone may work when you're ripping off a bandaid. But I've found that it doesn't work for most men when dealing with the tragedy and loss of businesses, reputations, and loved ones. When men are only ruthless, it's like ripping a man's arrow out and yelling at him to get back out on the battlefield. This "man up "strategy doesn't work; this isn't masculine care.

Warriors have heart and ruthlessness alone is heartless. It's when you combine the two that you create the environment for honesty, growth, and inspiration. The best example I have is when my dad sat on my bedside every day as a teenager. Without fail, he showed up and tried to help me get me out of bed and into class. Eventually, when the compassion alone wasn't cutting it, he threw a bucket of water on my head and changed my life. That experience was a literal wake up call for me and a vivid example of how the combination of ruthlessness and compassion plays a critical role in giving a fuck about another man.

Circle Up

In *Atomic Habits*, James Clear shares that one of the most important laws to behaviour change is to make it easy. He describes the law of least effort being, "Designing a life where doing the right thing is as easy as possible. "The entire purpose of this chapter is to normalize being able to ask for help. The best way I know how to make that action the easiest to do, is to find your men.

These are men you can talk to about anything. Your addictions, your insecurities, and even that time you shit your pants. These men are likely already in your life. And even if they're not, they're in Circle Up or maybe in your dance class. They could be a parent, a guardian, or a community leader you trust. Like I found when I launched Circle Up at the beginning of 2020, men all over the world are craving this conversation. They've been waiting for an opportunity to take off their mask in a safe space, take a deep breath, and honour their truth.

As you begin, or continue your journey, to establish and invest in these relationships; cherish them. If you've found a man you can be completely honest with about what you're struggling with, you're the exception, not the rule. In a study done by Prior Hospitals Group, they found that 40% of men in crisis won't talk to anyone, often because they feel like they have no one to turn to. Another study showed that men feel they have no one, or only one person, they'd feel comfortable talking to about their mental health. Do not allow that to be you or the men you care about.

We can choose a different path. We can learn from the men who struggled alone and honour their legacy. Our actions today represent the shift of consciousness we want to see for ourselves and for the men around us. We don't need more men that man up when their life gets tough. We need more men who give a fuck about each other. We don't need more men who're walking around wearing a mask. We need more men who're giving each other the space and permission to take it off and express themselves. And we definitely don't need more men who think their struggle means they're alone, because they're not.

While the past is the best indicator we have of future results, we can choose differently. Start with trusting one man. Then, another. Eventually, as we've already begun, we will make the most necessary action, of being honest and reaching out for help, the easy one. That is the work of masculine care and I'm excited to be in the trenches paving the way with you.

Circle Up!

San Marcos, Guatemala - June 2021

CHAPTER SUMMARY

Masculine care is about finding the fine line between ruthlessness and compassion. All compassion with no ruthlessness and we have our warriors walking around life without ever confronting their injuries and arrows from battle. All ruthlessness with no compassion, and we're perpetuating toxic masculinity conditioning. Neither of these approaches work in the case of men's mental health. One is all heart and no backbone. The other, all spine and no love. Ruthless compassion facilitates masculine relationships so that the action that matters most, normalizing help seeking behaviour during a mental health struggle, is the easiest action to take. The future of man up is Circle Up.

Resource Summary

Stay close to the resources, quotes, and thinkers you resonated most with in this chapter. Pay attention to what speaks to your heart. If you said to yourself, "I should check that out, "take action immediately.

1. **Men's Weekend - Sterling-institute.com - Justin Sterling**
2. **@thearminshafee - Instagram - Armin Shaffee**
3. *Shantaram* **- Gregory David Roberts**
4. *The Alchemist* **- Paulo Coelho**
5. **Advanced Forum - Landmark Worldwide**
6. *How To Change Your Mind: What The New Science of Psychedelics Teaches Us About Consciousness, Dying, Addiction, Depression, and Transcendence* **- Michael Pollen**
7. *Circle Up Podcast* **- Spotify - Jonathan Andrews**
8. *Daring Greatly* **- Brene Brown**
9. **Bethere.org - Jack.org**
10. *Atomic Habits* **- James Clear**
11. **Out of Your Mind -** Audible.com **- Alan Watts**

Self Reflection Opportunity

Once complete, move these notes to your phone. This will serve to summarize what you have learned, as well as ensure the resources, quotes, and ideas you personally resonated with most, are available at your fingertips.

Key points to remember (fill in here):

Who is a man in my life that I trust completely and can tell them anything and everything?

Who is a man in my life that I can take the risk to tip my mask with and begin the process of developing a masculine relationship with?

What is one idea from this chapter that will help me "set a better sail" in my own personal philosophy?

PART TWO
THE FUTURE OF "MAN UP"

CHAPTER SIX:

OFF THE COUCH AND ONTO THE BATTLEFIELD

"The thinker without paradox is like the lover without that feeling; a paltry mediocrity."

Soren Kierkegaard

There's No Such Thing As Dragons

The final idea that completes this book and my personal philosophy on men's mental health is that, as men, we need to man up. Now, you may be scratching your head at that and thinking "Didn't you just spend five chapters talking about the importance of not manning up? "Yes, I did. That said, hear me out. This missing element to the philosophy, this paradox, finally became clear to me in the most peculiar of places, in a children's book called *There's No Such Thing As A Dragon.* Recommended by Jordan Peterson, this profound book tells the story of the Bixbee family and the dragon that so quickly caused chaos in their home.

The story opens with, "Billy Bixbee was rather surprised when he woke up one morning and found a dragon in his room. It was a small dragon about the size of a kitten. The dragon wagged its tail happily when Billy patted his head. "Later, when Billy pointed out the dragon to his mother, she replied, "There's no such thing as a dragon! "When Billy was back alone in his room and the dragon again came close and wagged its tail, Billy didn't pet it. As the story goes, "If there's no such thing as something, it's silly to pat it on the head. "

The next thing they knew the dragon was the size of a dog. It grows larger and larger throughout the story the more and more it gets ignored. Eventually, it is the size of his mother, the size of their hall-way, and, finally, the size of their entire house. Billy then remarked, "I didn't know dragons grew so fast "and while his mother spent the entire morning cleaning the house, climbing in and out of the windows to get from room to room, she replied, ironically, "There's no such thing as a dragon! "

When Mr. Bixbee, Billy's dad, finally came home and asked how all this chaos happened, Billy said, "It was the dragon! "And before his mother could say there's no such thing, Billy added, "There is a dragon! "and patted it on the head. Again, it wagged its tail like it had in the opening scenes, and even faster than it had grown, it started getting smaller. On the concluding page, when the mother asked Billy why he thought it got so big, he ended this powerful children's story off by sharing, "I'm not sure... but I think it just wanted to be noticed. "

This story reminds me of a lot of masks, a concept we've explored in depth throughout this book, and how challenging it is to be honest about the dragons we face in our lives. It taught me that, like the weeds in a garden, what is ignored, grows and multiplies. That when we neglect what we fear and makes us uncomfortable, it only comes back fiercer and with more vigor later. The major lesson being, if something is nagging you, you better deal with it.

If there's something deficient in your personality, you're going to be happy that you did something about it today when it was the size of a kitten rather than wait five years for it to be so big that it takes over your life. Whatever that dragon is for you, addiction, trauma, or toxic beliefs about yourself and the world, you ought to face it. The time is now. It's time to man up.

By 'man up,' I do not mean it in our current understanding; to say take on your struggles alone or that the challenges you face aren't valid.

As you know from the first five chapters of this book, we're stronger together. You don't need to struggle and face these dragons in your life on your own. On the contrary, if you understand our philosophy at Circle Up, you know we got you. But you do need to face them. Both are true. Manning up and not manning up arrive mutually. One without the other is the same as asking for black without the white, the ying without the yang, or the masculine without the feminine.

The words 'man up' are loaded with baggage, as we explored in chapter one. That doesn't mean the idea is useless. The desired context in which it is typically used is in an attempt to help a man rise above his challenges. Unfortunately, it is almost never delivered, and/or received, in this desired way. Instead, it is typically received as an undermining of the challenges, addictions, and arrows at hand, as if a man should disregard them completely and move on. This approach doesn't work.

This is why Circle Up exists; to recondition 'man up' and to empower men through a new way of looking at masculinity and their mental health. The future of 'man up' is 'Circle Up.' We define 'manning up' through the context of finding the strength within yourself to ask for help. The courage to face your dragons, or become the type of man who trusts in himself and in his men so that he can drop his mask and be honest about his struggles. When I say, "We need to recondition our relationship with 'man up,' this is what I mean. It's simply a matter of context when you use the words.

Think back to the idea of masculine care and ruthless compassion we explored in the last chapter. All compassion with no ruthlessness and we have men walking around life without ever confronting their injuries and arrows from battle. These men become soft and allow doubt to cripple them. They're unable to take action and get out of their heads, too afraid to ever step back out on the battlefield. Most of these men will live their lives taking the easy path, and few, if any, will live their destiny and give their fullest gifts.

All ruthlessness with no compassion, the common use of 'man up' in our culture today, and we're perpetuating toxic masculinity conditioning. We spent the vast majority of this book exploring how those thoughts and ways of being don't work. In these cases, we raise lone wolves with no emotion, no empathy, and no heart. They may fight, but they fight alone. And when they struggle, they also struggle alone. In both cases, they live their lives feeling separated from other men. They're hard, but brittle. Willing to act, but only to survive, not be of service and to leave the world better than they found it.

Neither of these approaches work. One is all heart and no backbone. The other, all spine and no love. When we can't find the middle ground of ruthless compassion, of Circling Up, we have men suffering alone, contemplating whether life is worth it, and millions of them decidedly believing it is not. As Soren Kierkegaard, a prolific writer and intellectual, once wrote, "The thinker without paradox is like the lover without that feeling; a paltry mediocrity. "So if it feels like I'm contradicting myself now, know that it is because I intend to love you with my full truth.

More importantly, as your brother, I think of you highly enough to know that you can take it. Every idea up to this point was to share my belief that, no matter what you're going through, you are not alone. That, if you're suffering, you don't need to man up, you can Circle Up. And now I'm telling you, you also need to man up.

As a teenager struggling with my mental health, taking antidepressants, and feeling suicidal, my life didn't change until I did. I had all the love anyone could ask for around me from parents and those who cared, yes, but it was me who had to grab my balls and decide to get off the couch. I had to face my dragons and throw out the bongs and the weed and step into the gym. ☯[32] At the end of the day, I had to stop waiting for things to change, and instead, make it so.

---

32 ☯ **Philosophy Footnote:** *"You can't pay someone to do your push ups for you." - Jim Rohn*

Now that you know, without a shadow of a doubt, that you're not alone on this journey, it's time for you too, to be in action. To ask for help. To get off the couch. And it's time for you too, to do the things you know you need to do, but haven't. That is what manning up looks like from our point of view. Remember, it is doubt that kills the warrior. Manning up is nothing more than becoming the type of man who takes action in the face of his fears. Whether your dragon is a drug addiction, the tragic loss of a loved one, or any number of crippling fears that keep men off the battlefield and on the couch, it is now the time to face them.

Who can do this for you?

Only you can.

You are 100% responsible for your actions. There is no one else to blame. With that liberating truth in mind, I ask you, how much further along would you be today, if, instead of living in your head and standing inside of doubt, you manned up and faced your dragons? My final offering in service of helping you construct the castle of your dreams are the best tools and ideas I've implemented in my pursuit of becoming the type of man who faces his own dragons.

In becoming the type of man who has found his brothers and knows how and when to Circle Up and ask for help. Most importantly, the type of man who is on the battlefield taking consistent and bold steps towards the life of his dreams. ☯[33] With this chapter in your hands, you know the path. Actually walking it, right now, and consistently, is up to you.

REWIRED

Because the future of man up is Circle Up, we will refer to them as a single idea moving forward. Jim Rohn made the process of personal development and Circling Up the simplest. He said, "For things to

---

33 ☯ **Philosophy Footnote:** *"The difference between the people that 'do it' and the ones who don't is that the one group did it and the other didn't." - Iain Gabriel*

change, you need to change. "Now, I wasn't too receptive in my teenage years struggling with depression and addiction, but Jim Rohn somehow broke through to me. He said, "Unless you change how you are, you'll always have what you've got."

Looking at my life, terrified to get out of bed, let alone walk the hallways of my school, I realized he was right. He showed me there is no one else to blame. The school system wasn't going to change, the government wasn't going to change, my friends weren't going to change, and if none of these factors in my life were ever going to change, how would my life change? Jim made it crystal clear to me when he said, "When *you* change."

So, as a first step on this path to confronting dragons, overcoming addictions, and healing from the arrows of your past, I offer you Jim's greatest gift to me, when you change, everything will change for you. ☯[34] When you get better, everything will get better for you. My hope is that this truth is as liberating an insight for you as it was for me at seventeen years old. The big difference between hearing this today and hearing it almost a decade ago is that today, we now know the science of life change rather than simply the philosophy.

Because Iain loves great ideas, he's always reading and learning *something*. With enthusiasm, after virtually every single book he reads, he comes up to advocate I check it out. So much so, I decided to implement a philosophy filtering system, where I would only invest my time in reading or listening to any of his recommendations if he talked about it for more than a few weeks in a row. If he was still excited about the ideas, implementing the philosophy, and relating the impact it was having in his life after a couple weeks, I knew it was worth investing time into.

One of those mentors, who'd end up revealing the science behind the philosophy that Jim Rohn had taught me, was Joe Dispenza.

34 ☯ **Philosophy Footnote:** *"When you change the way you look at the world, the world you look at changes." - Iain Gabriel*

Iain read *Breaking The Habit Of Being Yourself*, and I could see that after a few weeks, it was having a dramatic positive impact on his life. Based on multiple additional recommendations from friends, and seeing firsthand Iain's life change for the better, I knew there was likely a deep reservoir of gems to be found in his work if I dared explore more. And there was.

At the beginning of 2021, I listened to Joe's program, *Rewired*, and found that he's now become a celebrity in the world of neuroscience, meditation, and behaviour change. Joe does a phenomenal job of bridging the gap of philosophy and spirituality with science. For analytical thinkers who want data, statistics, and proof that taking specific actions will improve their life, Joe is perfect.

The Science of Life Change

My biggest personal take away from the lectures was that no matter where you're starting from, you have the power to change your personal reality. Joe describes your personal reality, or the circumstances of your life, being shaped by, "Certain responses to stimulus repeated over time." Those responses to stimulus are who you are or your personality. So if you want to change your personal reality (your life circumstances), you must begin by changing your responses to stimulus, aka your personality. That idea made sense to me, so I dove in deeper.

Like we discussed in chapter one, if you can change your thoughts and the way you look at the world, or as Jim put it, "the sail on your sailboat," the direction of your life will change. Jim used to tell the story of how in the first five years of his economic life, he wound up broke and didn't have two dollars to his name. The next five, he was a millionaire. What changed? It was his thinking that changed. His personal philosophy. And, therefore, the direction of his life changed. The same thing happened to me when I was in high school.

For three years, I was planting the seeds in the garden of my mind of fear, doubt, and why the world was cruel and unfair. In the next three years, I found personal development and my life changed. I started to believe in ideas like, "You can have more than you've got if you become more than you are, ""Success is not to be pursued, it's to be attracted by the person you become, "and "Life doesn't get better by chance, it gets better by change. "Jim helped kickstart my personal development journey, and when my thinking changed, I started to change. So can you.

As mentioned, Joe Dispenza's program *Rewired*, connected science to these philosophies and demonstrated that your personality begins at the level of thinking. *Rewired* teaches that you have about 60,000-70,000 thoughts a day. The research also shows that 90% of those thoughts are the same as the day before. So, the question for us becomes: what's the likelihood of something happening differently in our lives if 90% of our thoughts, conscious or unconscious, are the same as the day before? Highly unlikely.

Joe shared that the same thoughts will always lead to the same choices. The same choices will always lead to the same experiences. The same experiences will always create the same emotions. And now, just like how doubt leads to inaction, which leads to more doubt, this process of creating your personality is also cyclical. Those emotions drive the same thoughts and the cycle repeats itself, rooting us more deeply into our current identity and personality.

Who you are becomes a set of memorized behaviours, automatic habits, emotional reactions, beliefs, perceptions, and attitudes that function like the programming on a computer. If you're mindful, that programming will put you in a position to thrive and live a life of abundance and love. If you're not, your lack of mindfulness about your responses to stimuli in your life, or your personality, may be leading you towards hell on earth.

As we discussed in chapter one, you can think of your personal reality as the fruit you pick at harvest time and your personality being the seeds you plant in the spring. The fruit, or your personal reality, is just a result. It's a symptom of a seed you've been planting with your personality and the person you've become. I'll repeat Jim when he said, "Whatever you reap is what you've sown. "In order for us to harvest the fruits of a new personal reality, we must first address the seed.

If you want to live in a new house, have a better body, or become the type of person who acts in the face of fear, then you have to start changing your personality. Most people try to create a new life with the same personality, but Joe's research, Jim's philosophical prose, and just plain common sense, reveal to us this doesn't work. In order to change, you need to change. You literally need to become someone else.

What this means is simple. Joe describes your personal reality or the circumstances of your life as being shaped by "Certain responses to stimulus repeated over time. "Those responses to stimulus are who you are or your personality. So, if you want to change your personal reality (your life circumstances), all you need to do is change the way you habitually respond to stimuli in your environment. It's that simple.

This whole chapter is dedicated to facilitating this focus as effortlessly as possible.

A final note before offering actionable insight as to how to go about changing your personality is that Joe's research shows, by the time you are thirty-five years old, 95% of who you are, these computer-like programmed automated habits and memorized behaviours, become rigid and inflexible. This is likely where axioms like, "You can't teach an old dog new tricks, "although untrue, came from. For this reason, therefore, in addition to the ideas outlined in this book, readers above thirty-five may benefit greatly from exploring psychedelics as a modality for life-change.

An analogy I find useful, relating the possibilities of psychedelics with these automated habits and memorized behaviours, is to think of your life like travelling down a snowy ski slope. The decisions we make daily activate neural networks and wiring in our brains that can be thought of as creating grooves in the snow as you ski down the exact same path day after day. With every daily repetition, the wiring strengthens and so does the depth and width of the groove we're making as we ski.

If you try to change your life, let's say after a decade of alcoholism or of smoking cigarettes, it's very difficult to ski down a new path without falling right back into the automated habits and memorized behaviours that created these deep grooves. What psychedelics seem to offer these people, is a full day of hard falling fresh new snow. With the grooves temporarily filled, possibility exists. Decisions or ways of being that seemed obvious the day before are now suddenly questioned as to their logic and personal benefit.

Are these actions really the person I want to become? For many people, they realize no and are able to change. For those interested in learning more, a read by bestselling author and globally respected journalist, Michael Pollen titled *How To Change Your Mind: What The New Science of Psychedelics Teaches Us About Consciousness, Dying, Addiction, Depression, and Transcendence* may offer the perfect starting point. Research out of some of our most respected universities globally are demonstrating the efficacy for these powerful consciousness expanding drugs to reduce or eliminate depression, anxiety, and PTSD symptoms as well as help those suffering from addiction.

They are also a tool I've used personally in the pursuit of my better mental health to great positive benefit.

Allow Your Vision To Pull You

Why is any of this important? Because the science of rewiring our brains, and therefore, our lives, shows us that if we're going to have any chance of becoming a new man, the first step, as we explored in depth in chapter one, is awareness. The next step, as Joe suggests, is to break the habit of being yourself. Fortunately, you already laid all the groundwork for this life change in chapter three. You brought forth the vision for your future and we explored and answered questions like:

- **What does your new future look like?**
- **What are you doing?**
- **Who are you with?**
- **What habits do you practice?**
- **Who are you being?**
- **What feelings are associated with this new life?**

If you followed along with this exercise from chapter three (and I encourage you to go back and follow along if you haven't you lazy jerk), you've begun the process of changing your personal reality by developing a mantra rooted in your vision for your new future. This mantra is a thought-seed that has the potential, if nourished and cared for, to manifest a new brilliant and abundant harvest in your life.

This exact creative process is what we used to take Circle Up from an idea to a world class personal development opportunity for men. Instead of being limited by our inherited context and conditioning surrounding men's mental health and masculinity, we created the context that:

- **Every man has mental health and no man struggles alone. Don't man up, Circle Up.**

It's from this context that we make decisions. It's from this way of looking at masculinity that we take action. And it's from this possibility, rooted in our vision of the future, that we're changing the way we think, feel, and act on our mental health. Today, like I hope you will choose to do, I am using this process for my own life.

In chapter two, we discussed masks and I shared my personal journey with my physical health. After my injury, I created a new personal reality for my life based on thoughts, experiences, feelings, and actions that were rooted in fear, dishonesty, and mistrust of myself. My predominant thought-seeds were that I was broken. I believed that I'd never be able to regain my strength and athleticism. Those thoughts quite literally created my own prison. Like how James Allen wrote in *As A Man Thinketh*, "As a man thinketh in his heart, so shall he be."

I am on this journey with you. Through this process of creating a vision of my future from possibility, I now have the key to unlock the prison doors that I myself created with my thoughts. You can do the same for your circumstances and your personal reality. The new mantra I've generated is rooted in the vision of myself competing in Olympic weightlifting, snatching a barbell over my head. ☯[35] While a lift like that would likely cripple me today, through the process of changing my thoughts and taking actions based on my new vision for the future, I will bring it forth. The new thought-seed I am planting is:

"I am grateful for my relaxed, strong, and playful; mind, body, and spirit."

What is your new thought-seed? Refer back to our exercise from chapter three and write it out here. This thought may need refinement based on the additional learnings we've explored since that chapter. I encourage you to make these adjustments, as the person you want to become, and the life you want to live, changes over time.

Your mantra here:

This exercise is the foundation of changing your thoughts and your personality. It is also the practical application of Jim Rohn's idea of learning to set a better sail. Moving forward, all of your decisions,

35 ☯ **Philosophy Footnote:** *"Cherish your visions; cherish your ideals; cherish the music that stirs in your heart, the beauty that forms in your mind, the loveliness that drapes your purest thoughts, for out of them will grow all delightful conditions, all heavenly environment; of these, if you will remain true to them, your world will at last be built." - James Allen*

associations, and daily actions, will be anchored by this vision so as to help you course-correct your personality over time. Eventually leading you to a life that was once just a dream. This process, as Joe Dispensa says, "is your experiment with destiny."

Key Point: Apply Auto-suggestion to facilitate your new life.

In Napoleon Hill's *Think And Grow Rich*, the most popular personal development text of all time, he interviewed over 500 of the world's richest and most successful men, like Andrew Carnegie, Henry Ford, and Charles M. Schwab. From that research, he generated a concept called Auto-suggestion that you can apply now in allowing your subconscious mind to aid you in manifesting the life of your dreams. Auto-suggestion is a self-induced suggestion, which you can use to guide your thoughts, feelings and actions. Instead of leaving your 60,000 thoughts a day to chance, Auto-suggestion will help you align your thinking with your new personal reality as often as humanly possible.

Grab your phone. We will use it now to create a reminder to message you every day, as many times as you'd like. Auto-suggest the direction you're headed:

1. **Open up your reminders app**
2. **Write your new thought-seed, such as, "I am grateful for my relaxed, strong, and playful mind, body, and spirit."**
3. **Create a reminder so that your phone messages you this at least once a day ☯[36]**

Jim Rohn calls this daily queue, "The silent seminar. "Every morning at 8 a.m., my reminder sends me this message and I let it speak to me throughout the day. This is critical because we get busy, distracted,

36 ☯ **Philosophy Footnote:** *"Of the same vain, and as per Jonathan's recommendation, something I have as a daily notification reminder on my phone is 'What is my context?'" - Iain Gabriel*

and life happens. Additionally, as Joe's research alludes to, all of your automatic habits and memorized behaviour act as a sort of gravitational pull in the groove of how you've always done things. Therefore, making a mantra but not using it daily as a tool to see if your decisions are in alignment with this new vision, is like buying a lottery ticket and leaving your financial future up to chance.

Don't be that guy. Instead, Auto-suggestion facilitates that every day, no matter what, you will be reminded of your intention. Additionally, if you'd like to take this a step further you can make cue cards with your new intention and put one on your bathroom mirror, inside of your car, or anywhere you will see it daily. A good friend of mine, Ally Salama, who is the Mental Health Ambassador for the Middle East, uses this process to great effect.

Every time I go to his house, he has his most important goal or chief aim up on a whiteboard. For over a year, he had "Forbes 30 Under 30 "written on his bathroom wall and surprise, surprise, he made it happen. Ally is a Forbes 30 Under 30. And he is one of the truest examples in my life of the idea that we're only limited by our own imaginations. This Auto-suggestion, as Napoleon Hill and Ally have demonstrated, has worked for history's most successful men and will act as a reminder, if you let it, to ensure that no matter how busy life gets, you will be thinking about your new future, daily. Do this now.

You now know exactly where you want to go and that, for things to change for you, you need to change. These next steps, as you can imagine, are challenging and uncomfortable. Embrace them. If they weren't uncomfortable, you wouldn't grow. If there was no doubt, you wouldn't be on the battlefield. This discomfort is a necessary part of the process of bringing forth your new life.

Furthermore, remember that this is the battlefield you've chosen! This vision isn't just some set of circumstances that fell into your lap or that you stumbled into. This is your life. This is your dream. Be excited! As Jim Rohn said, "If there's one thing to get excited about, it's your ability to make yourself do the necessary things to get a desired result, to turn the negative into success."

FUCK IT

Now that you're reminded of where you're headed, rooted in science, I offer you a second, totally unscientific approach that I believe connects poeticaly to the ideas we've explored here.

In October of 2019, I flew to Europe to party at the Amsterdam Music Festival and surprise Iain in the middle of his three week Euro trip. On my eight hour flight across the sea, I was compelled to pull out my journal and write about the biggest battle a man faces in his lifetime; the one between his own two ears. ☯[37] Thousands of years ago, this mental battle would have gotten us killed physically, and, today, it's responsible for the slow spiritual death of countless millions of men.

This is the letter I wrote to myself:

Imagine you're standing on the battlefield defending your homeland. Brothers to your left and right, sword in one hand, shield in the other. From only a hundred yards away, you hear drums, war cries, and the deafening footsteps of enemy warriors. With an army charging at you and adrenaline coursing through your body, you tightly grip your sword, put one foot in front of the other, and stare death in the face. With chaos in every direction, you see the perfect opportunity to strike, but you hesitate. In that split second of hesitation, you feel hot steel rip through your shoulder, your own blood gushing onto the grass under your feet, and your vision blurring as it all fades away.

What am I talking about here?

---

37 ☯ **Philosophy Footnote:** *"The mass of men live lives of quiet desperation." - Henry David Thoreau*

This story, and that battle of a lifetime, is about doubt.

In my Men's Weekend, our seminar leader, Justin Sterling, described that 1,000 years ago, it was doubt that killed the warrior. A split second hesitation meant the difference between life and death. Today, while the stakes aren't as high, and the immediate consequences of doubt are not as obvious, doubt is continuing to wreak havoc on men and their mental health. When I look back on my time as a teenager, where my confidence and self-esteem were at an all time low, I can attribute it to inaction.

I now see clearly the truth in Jim Rohn's words when he said, "The only thing worse than the wrong direction is no direction."

When I allowed doubt to creep into my life, it zapped my ambition and landed me crashing on the couch. I was full of anxiety, addictions, and excuses for why my life wasn't working out. And because I was in the basement, I had no hope, no light, and no direction. ☯[38]

Doubt is everywhere. You know you deserve a raise at work, but you're fearful of your boss's reaction so you never ask for it. You see a cute girl and really want to ask for her number, but you're too scared of rejection so you don't even say hi. Or maybe you're like me and wanted to write a book, start a business, or make a change in your life, but were afraid of being judged and ridiculed so it remained dormant as a draft for six months (circa 2019 before I committed to finishing this book).

---

38 ☯ **Philosophy Footnote:** *"Sit or walk as you will, but whatever you do, don't wobble." - Alan Watts.*

If you're like me, you can look back on countless "woulda, coulda, shoulda" moments when doubt crept in and you let it take you off course, the wind out of your sails, and kill the warrior inside of you. ☯[39] Fortunately, the men who've come before us have faced this internal battle for thousands of years and developed a tried-and-tested action plan for facing our dragons, getting onto the battlefield, and manning up.

It's two words: Fuck It! ☯[40]

The first time I remember consciously using this philosophy was in the spring of 2019. I was in a bad head space about women and relationships. I had just broken up with my long-term girlfriend of six years and rejection from women had become one of my dragons. That fear was taking over my life. I remember the day it all changed.

I was dancing down the stairs at the ST George subway platform in Toronto, headphones in, listening to AC Slater's Fly Kicks. There were about forty people waiting for trains as the song was building to one of my favourite electronic music drops of all time. I was compelled to dance and so I did. Harder than anyone should in the middle of the subway, I left it all on the "dance floor" that day. As I regained my composure and became aware again of my surroundings, I saw a cute girl out of the corner of my eye laughing at me.
99 times out of 100, I see that good looking woman after what I just did, and I

---

39 ☯ **Philosophy Footnote:** *"It's been said that the greatest inventions, the best songs, books, etc. that have ever been conceived in human history reside in the cemetery, with all the dreams that stayed as such." - Iain Gabriel*

40 ☯ **Philosophy Footnote:** *"Don't let your dreams be dreams! Just do it!" - Shia Lebouf*

would quickly look away, get on the train, and, filled with shame, hope to never see her again. But not on that day. On that day, in that moment, I saw her laugh at me and just said, "fuck it." I walked straight up to her and said, "My name's Jonathan, I think you're super cute. Who are you?" She went on to be one of the most important women in my life.

She helped me to shape my character and fostered in me a desire to be a better man. That memory will be forever seared into my mind because I didn't act that day as a result of being full of confidence, or because I was sure she'd be into me—in fact, I was pretty sure she thought I was an idiot. I acted that day because I chose to. That day made me realize that I've always had that choice.

It made me wonder how many opportunities for joy, personal growth, and love I'd missed out on over the course of my life by letting fear overcome me. It made me realize that no one's ever held me back from accomplishing any of my dreams other than me. Every time I've listened to the voices of doubt, I became more of a man who let doubt hold him back and less of a man who took action in spite of fear.

"Fuck It" Is Broscience That Works

These two ideas paired together, Joe Diespenza's science backed research on changing your personal reality and Justin Sterling's keep it simple stupid protocol for decision making, make magic. Or Broscience.

However you position it, it works!

Like the "If this, then that "stress triggers we explored in chapter four, you can use "fuck it "to pattern-interrupt your typical fear, doubt, and discomfort responses. If your personality, as Joe puts it, is your responses to stimulus repeated over time, then all we need to do, as men looking to bringforth our new vision, is to say "fuck it "any time we are presented with an oportunity to move towards that new life. Do not underestimate the power of a single "fuck it. "

There are dozens of "fuck it "opportunities sprinkled throughout your day, and success, as Jim Rohn pointed out, "is nothing more than a few simple disciplines practiced every day. "To demonstrate how a single "fuck it "holds the potential to shift your personality, consider a small degree of change in a plane's trajectory at takeoff.

In James Clear's *Atomic Habits*, he says, "If the pilot was to make only a 3.5 degree change in direction south for a plane flying from Los Angeles to New York City, the plane would end up in Washington DC instead of New York City. "As you can see, a change barely noticeable when taking off leads you hundreds of miles away from your intended destination.

He argued that our success isn't a matter of dramatic life changes, but, instead, the man you are versus the man you could be is the result of 1% changes in your daily decisions. This philosophy aligns perfectly with Jim Rohn as he continued his success equation by offering it's flip side. "Failure "he said, "is simply a few errors in judgement repeated every day. "For example, if the new intention you've set is to be strong and lean and so you say "fuck it "to an apple a day instead of a Hershey bar a day, each "fuck it "casts a vote in the direction of the man you've always wanted to be.

On the other hand, if your current personality persists and you choose a Hershey bar every day instead of an apple, you're actively casting votes in the trajectory of your current personal reality. By using "fuck it "and interrupting your memorized behaviours and automatic responses to the stimulus that make you feel doubt and fear, you're becoming a new man. You're changing the habit of being yourself.

Don't overthink this. Next time you feel like eating that cookie, but your new vision is of a man who is lean and full of energy and vitality, say "fuck it "and toss the box in the garbage. That's how "fuck it " works. That's how your life change works. As weeks and months pass, you'll have casted more and more votes for the man you've always wanted to be and you *will* see progress. Eventually, the automatic habits and memorized behaviours that once acted as a ball and shackle to your leg, keeping you in the basement full of anxiety and doubt, will become the very same habits that free your body, mind, and spirit.

THE TRAGIC COSMIC JOKE

If you're anything like me, you want direction that is specific and actionable. So instead of leaving the changes you want to make in your personality to chance, let's close this chapter by applying a concept I learned from Justin Sterling on practicing daily disciplines.

Justin called this process the Tragic Cosmic Joke and explained that, as men, we're either committed or addicted. He said, "The degree to which you are committed is the degree to which you are not addicted. " Or, in the case of men who are struggling, the opposite is typically true, "The degree to which you are addicted is the degree to which you are not committed. "He said that the most important question a man can ask himself is "What am I committed to? "

Once we know what we're committed to as a man, we can surrender to our commitment. Commitment is a powerful tool for men because when it is coupled with the appropriate daily discipline, it will shape and mold our character. The Ownership Icon we use at Circle Up teaches that:

"As your ownership in your mission increases, the needs of the task start to shape and mold you to suit it. If decisiveness is necessary, then he will develop that trait. If sensitivity to emotion is needed, he will acquire that ability. If the purpose or task that he has chosen is worthy, honorable, and true to his commitment, then the evolution of his character will be enhanced by surrendering fully to his commitment. "

Therefore, we will now take your new vision for the future and couple it with a simple daily discipline so as to refine and mold your personality to suit your desired personal reality. I can personally credit this exercise, and its consistent application, to helping me learn how to play guitar, speak Spanish, and write this book all in the last couple years. Let's do it together now.

Self-Reflection Opportunity

Step one: Identify an addiction

An addiction is something in control of you versus something that you control. So, bring to mind your mantra and commitment to your new life. What behaviour do you express daily that will actively get in the way for you to manifest this new personal reality?

> **1.1 Brainstorm all of your "failure actions" - the behaviours you express when you feel at your worst**

For example, I have chosen to identify my personality when I was struggling in High School in order to give me insight into what I do, and how I choose to live, when my judgement is poor. These are your actions that lead to failure or as Jim Rohn suggested, your "few errors in judgement repeated daily "behaviours.

My Example

The times I've felt at my lowest I consistently chose:

- To eat processed foods like fast food, candies, pancakes with syrup every morning, chocolate bars, dairy products, and other junk food
- To stay up late watching TV, porn, or YouTube videos on my laptop
- To sleep past my alarm and not wake up until noon consistently
- To skip my classes and show up late
- To listen to music that makes me feel angry or sad

- To quit sports like trampoline and skip hockey games and practice
- To spend most of the day inside my house
- To play videogames on my Xbox for multiple hours daily
- To smoke weed from the minute I woke up till it was time to go to bed
- To isolate myself from friends, family and community
- To think of myself as worthless and incapable
- To allow myself to go multiple days without showering

YOUR TURN

The times I've felt at my lowest I consistently chose:

-
-
-
-
-
-
-
-
-
-

1.2 Choose which behaviour, substance, or way of being is the addiction you desire to replace with a discipline

This exercise is designed to help you identify which part of your current personality is in control of you versus you being in control of it. From there, we can replace the addiction with discipline, change our lives, and become new people. This exercise is the practical application of Carl Jung's idea that "Until you make the unconscious conscious, it will direct your life and you will call it fate."

My Example

The addiction I choose to replace is: Smoking weed.

My Why: I allow weed to control me and I will often "wake and bake," preventing me from feeling focused on my work, in my physical health and exercise, and for important moments.

Your Turn

The addiction I choose to replace is:

My Why:

Key Point: Drugs and other forms of common addictions are not inherently good or bad.

Remember these behaviours aren't inherently good or bad—most anything is doable in moderation. I love weed. Marijuana has led to some of the most important conversations and creative breakthroughs I've ever had. There are few things more fun to me than to share a spliff with friends and listen and dance to good music.

The challenge is not that weed or other substances are inherently bad, although there are many that are proven to be much more destructive and neurotoxic than others, the challenge is that I am not in control. This exercise is not to make yourself wrong, it's to simply identify a behaviour that

has gotten control of you and become part of your personality that is also not in alignment with the direction of your new personal reality.

Step two: Create a discipline that replaces the addiction

Do not misinterpret this as stopping or resisting the addiction. This is a mistake. "What you resist, "as network marketing legend George Zalucki reminds us, "will persist. "Instead, focus 100% of your attention and energy on the discipline to be implemented. Your commitment will automatically diminish the addiction as the degree to which you are committed is the degree to which you're not addicted.

2.1 Brainstorm your "success actions" - all of the behaviours you express when you feel at your best

For example, I chose to identify my personality when my energy levels, enthusiasm for life, and sense of purpose were at all time highs. These behaviours give me insight into what I do and how I choose to live when I am walking the path to the man I've always wanted to be. These are your success actions. As Jim Rohn suggested, your "few simple disciplines practiced every day "behaviours.

MY EXAMPLE

The times I've felt at my best I consistently chose:

- To meditate daily
- To workout with resistance training daily
- To walk multiple times a day with as much skin as possible exposed to the sun
- To eat whole foods like fruits, vegetables, quality protein and avoid virtually all processed food following the guidelines from Michael Pollen's *Food Rules* book
- To write gratitude in my journal daily

- To call a friend or to remind someone I love them daily
- To work on a project or an idea that aligned with my purpose and the direction I want to take my life daily
- To read or learn something new and exciting to me every day
- To listen to music that inspires me
- To get at least 7-8 hours of quality sleep every night

YOUR TURN

The times I've felt at my best I consistently chose:

2.2 Choose which behaviour will become your new daily discipline for the next thirty days

This exercise is designed to help you identify the disciplines that, if practiced daily, will shape your personality and act like a magnet pulling your new personal reality towards you.

MY EXAMPLE

The daily discipline I choose to implement is: Every day for thirty days after my morning walk, I will complete my workout program in my home.

Key Point: The degree to which you're successful with your new daily discipline will be based on the degree to which you're specific.

Make sure your discipline includes when, where, with who, and for how long you're committed. The more ambiguity, the more likely you will bullshit yourself and justify why you can skip a day or wait till tomorrow.

*Notice that I have answered for:

How long - thirty days in a row

When - after my morning walk

With who - in solitude, alone

Where - in my home

Answering, "workout "or "workout daily "is a recipe for confusion and inaction. Set yourself up for success by making it simple and specific.

Your Turn

The daily discipline I choose to implement for the next thirty days is:

How long -

When -

With who -

Where -

Step three: Choose a compelling incentive structure (consequences and rewards)

In the same way that many effective workout programs involve both push and pull days, an effective commitment includes both consequences and rewards. Consequences push you while rewards pull you towards remaining disciplined and consistent.

3.1 Consequences

Consequences can manifest in the form of cold showers, doing push ups, and even public embarrassment like singing "I'm a little teapot " in the middle of Walmart. The importance here is to remember that a consequence is not a punishment. As men, you've likely noticed that not only do we fuck up, but we fuck up big and we fuck up often.

You're not a bad boy or wrong for breaking a streak or falling prey to addiction. You are, however, out of integrity. As a man, you are your word. You are what you say you're going to do. Therefore, if you want to garner respect and develop trust with other men and yourself, you can leverage consequences to become aware of when you break your word and to help you take your commitments and your honour as a man more seriously.

I like to think of my integrity and honour like water on the floor as a result of a leaky bucket. The more integrity I have, the smaller the hole in the bucket and the less of a mess I make. The more honour I have, the quicker I clean it up and get back into action without slipping and hurting myself because of my own lack of integrity.

It's virtually impossible to have perfect integrity all the time. Especially when you dream big, are living at your edge, and expanding towards a new personal reality. Our focus here is to use consequences that we self-generate in order to clean up the metaphorical mess we make, to get out of our heads, and to get back on the battlefield.

MY EXAMPLE

If I break my streak, my consequence will be: I will restart from day one and take a ten minute extremely cold shower (ouch).

YOUR TURN

If I break my streak, my consequence will be:

Key Point: Effective consequences make you uncomfortable.

Like mine above, it should be uncomfortable and painful enough that you would rather the discomfort of maintaining your discipline over having to do the consequence. In that sense, it pushes you towards your goal.

3.2 Rewards

When you hit milestones on your daily discipline, celebrate. How will you reward yourself for maintaining a seven day, fifteen day, and thirty day commitment to your new life? ☯[41]

41 ☯ *Philosophy Footnote: "Celebration is a rite of passage, and it honours the sacrifices you made, and renews and inspires strength to set further targets." - Iain Gabriel*

MY EXAMPLE

1. Seven day streak celebration – I will go to the local bakery and buy three of the most delicious-looking desserts on display.
2. 15 day streak celebration – I will take myself out for a steak dinner and a glass of red wine.
3. 30 day streak celebration – I will call or hangout with a friend and smoke a fat spliff.

YOUR TURN

1. **Seven day streak celebration - I will:**

2. **Fifteen day streak celebration - I will:**

3. **Thirty day streak celebration - I will:**

Key Point: Both consequences and rewards should be proportional to the discipline being consistently applied.

Similarly to how consequences push you away from screwing up, rewards should be compelling enough to pull you towards completing your commitment. For example, if I finish thirty days in a row of my discipline, a reasonable reward is a well deserved joint with a buddy. It is not, however, proportional to the discipline, to go on an all-expense-paid three week vacation because I worked out for thirty days.

Ensure that you're choosing both consequences and rewards that reasonably match the discipline. If you find yourself making commitments that you aren't keeping, check that both the consequences you've established and the rewards you're looking forward to are compelling. The point of making and keeping commitments is to develop a strong relationship with your word and to diminish addictions in your life. A man who does what he says he will do, consistently, and to the best of his ability, is a man you can trust and a man on the path of becoming the man he's always wanted to be.

Step four: Be accountable

By having a system for consequence and reward, you're already accountable to yourself. However, you can dramatically increase your odds of consistently taking action if you tell someone else about your discipline. You can use a man you trust, your Circle Up men's team, or anyone who you can count on to be honest with you. Either way, a daily message to an accountability partner that you've completed your discipline will make you less likely to buy your own bullshit and fuck this up.

My example

I am choosing to stay accountable by: Using my buddy on my Circle Up men's team as well as my men's team group chat to communicate the completion of my discipline every day for the first thirty days.

I will also post an instagram story every day at the end of my workout tagging @projectcircleup with the hashtag #circleupdailydisciplinechallenge

Your Turn

I am choosing to stay accountable by:

Key Point: Enjoy your friend's criticism.

A powerful lesson from David Deita's book *The Way Of The Superior Man: A Spiritual Guide to Mastering the Challenges of Women, Work, and Sexual Desire* is to enjoy your friend's criticism. I've learned throughout my life that keeping my word and having integrity is not a question of right or wrong. Rather, integrity is a question of workability. It works in life to do what you say you're going to do in your relationships, at work, and with yourself. While foreign to most people, by seeing integrity through the lense of what works and what doesn't versus what's right or wrong, a man no longer needs to hide out when he fucks up. He doesn't need to engage his ego with his men and protect himself with his mask.

If you have created a trusting, confidential space with your Circle Up men's team, you can bring your fuck ups, dishonourable actions, and broken agreements to your men. Use these spaces of accountability to be honest. Honesty will help you identify who you are so you know the gap between that man and the man you've always wanted to be.

Furthermore, as David Deita says, "Your close men friends should be willing to challenge your mediocrity by suggesting a concrete action you can perform that will pop you out of your rut, one way or the other. And you must be willing to offer them brutal honesty, in the same way, if you are all to grow."

Sometimes, we're blind to where we're out of integrity or dropping the ball on our commitments, but more often than that, we bullshit ourselves. Choose to be held accountable by friends who're challenging themselves and facing their own fears. "Men of this kind, "as David says, "can love you without protecting you from the necessary confrontation with reality that your life involves. "

Follow along with the prompts outlined in my example to create your own one-page daily discipline challenge. Outline your daily action plan in the following order:

- **Your vision for the future or your new commitment**
- **The addiction to be replaced**
- **The daily discipline to be implemented**
- **Your chosen consequence**
- **Your chosen rewards**
- **Your chosen accountability structure**
- **A thirty day commitment tracker to be crossed off after each successful completion of the discipline. Keep the streak going! Build that chain of X's and be proud of each day and each moment you choose your new life**
- **A quote that you can read each day that inspires you**

Jonathan's Daily Discipline Challenge Example

"I am grateful for my relaxed, strong, and playful mind, body, and spirit."

1. **The addiction I choose to replace is:** Smoking weed
2. **The daily discipline I choose to implement is:** Every day, for thirty days, after my morning walk, I will complete my workout program in my home.
3. **If I break my streak, my consequence will be:** I will restart from day one and take a ten minute extremely cold shower.
4. **As a reward, when I complete:**
    a. Seven day streak celebration – I will go the local bakery and buy three of the most delicious looking desserts on the display
    b. Fifteen day streak celebration – I will take myself out for a steak dinner and a glass of red wine
    c. Thirty day streak celebration – I will call or hangout with a friend and smoke a fat spliff
5. **I am choosing to stay accountable by:** Using my buddy on my men's team, my men's team group chat, and a daily instagram story with #circleupdailydisciplinechallenge to communicate the completion of my discipline everyday for the first thirty days.

Commitment Tracker

Day 1	Day 2	Day 3	Day 4	Day 5	Day 6	Day 7
Day 8	Day 9	Day 10	Day 11	Day 12	Day 13	Day 14
Day 15	Day 16	Day 17	Day 18	Day 19	Day 20	Day 21
Day 22	Day 23	Day 24	Day 25	Day 26	Day 27	Day 28
Day 29	Day 30					

"Success is nothing more than a few simple disciplines practiced every day; while failure is simply a few errors in judgement, repeated every day. It is the accumulative weight of our disciplines and our judgements that lead us to either fortune or failure."

Jim Rohn

#CircleUpDailyDisciplineChallenge (your turn)

"

1. The addiction I choose to replace is:

2. The daily discipline I choose to implement is:

3. If I break my streak, my consequence will be:

4. As a reward, when I complete:

    a. Seven day streak celebration -
    b. Fifteen day streak celebration -
    c. Thirty day streak celebration -

5. I am choosing to stay accountable by:

COMMITMENT TRACKER

Day 1	Day 2	Day 3	Day 4	Day 5	Day 6	Day 7
Day 8	Day 9	Day 10	Day 11	Day 12	Day 13	Day 14
Day 15	Day 16	Day 17	Day 18	Day 19	Day 20	Day 21
Day 22	Day 23	Day 24	Day 25	Day 26	Day 27	Day 28
Day 29	Day 30					

“

Yesterday You Said Tomorrow

If you're waiting for motivation to strike before you begin this process, don't. If your current personality reflects the type of man who's more likely to sit on the couch than to be on the battlefield, you may wait your whole life. When I first started writing this book, I dreaded every session.

Why?

Well, firstly, I had no writing discipline prior, so anything beyond nothing was more than I was used to. And secondly, I was making it too challenging for myself. Initially, I committed to an hour of writing a day. And while compared to a professional writer, that's child's play, to me, it seemed like an insurmountable obstacle.

I quickly found that all I needed to do to feel motivated to write was to sit down and write (lol). If it seems too good to be true, you'll be pleasantly surprised. Tim Ferriss' advice for writers is to commit to two crappy pages a day. James Clear made this concept more concrete to me when he explained the importance of making your new discipline as easy as possible. He shares the story of an overweight man who desperately wanted to lose weight and had tried all sorts of exercise programs that never stuck. Finally, he decided to take James' advice to make it easy and everything changed for him. He would drive to the gym every day on his way to work, but instead of working out, he would simply walk inside, look around, and then get back in his car and drive himself to the office.

How did this change his life?

This man ritualized the habit of going to the gym. After a few weeks of ingraining this new habit he says to himself, "Jesus, if I'm going to come to the gym every day, I might as well workout a little bit. " So he did. He started with a five-ten minute workout and when that became too easy for him, he progressed a bit more. By starting small and making the early stages of his life change so easy he couldn't fail, he eventually went on to lose over 100 pounds.

I think about this story a lot as I consult with myself and the men in Circle Up looking to improve their mental health. This is why we can't wait for motivation or the perfect moment to get started. The brain wants to conserve energy. It is much more likely to choose your current personality over something that requires effort. Therefore, as the man who spent weeks walking into the gym without a single workout demonstrated, in the beginning, it's more important to get off the couch and onto the battlefield than it is to slay dragons when you get there.

The early stages of life change are about facing your dragons, not slaying them.

In the beginning is when you will experience the biggest barriers to action. The monkeys will tell you that you need to have the perfect plan before you start or the perfect book before you publish. Unfortunately, this approach doesn't work. Having the perfect plan doesn't make you successful, taking action does. If you take consistent action towards the intention you set, you will make mistakes, but you will also learn and grow. George Zalucki, one of the most successful network marketing professionals of all time, ingrained in me to "Do the thing and you shall have the power."

What's the easiest way to have the power?

Do the thing!

What's the easiest way to do the thing?

As we've discovered, it's to make your new daily discipline easy.

Make it so easy, make the barrier of entry so small, that you cannot fail. Let everyone else struggle and strife to change their lives. Not you. Take the easy road. Choose a daily discipline where you're interrupting the pattern of your old personality while simultaneously laying the foundations, and neural networks, for your new life with an action that's so easy you can't fail. Inch by inch, you can build on top of the new discipline, creating a brand new personality, and, therefore, in the process, a brand new personal reality.

Circle Up

Everything about this chapter was designed to get you on the battlefield. Manning up, or what we will now refer to as Circling Up, is about gathering the strength to face your addictions, your arrows, and your dragons. But do not rush or be overly concerned about slaying them just yet. That will come in due time.

At Circle Up, we teach that becoming the type of warrior who slays dragons takes decades of commitment, persistence, and discipline. Becoming the type of man who gets off the couch and takes action in the face of his doubt and fear, however, takes a single decision. Your daily decisions are either moving you closer to the Castle of our dreams, or further from it. All you can do in your pursuit of the man you've always wanted to be is to make the next choice the right choice.

Who can do this for you?

Only you can.

As we discussed, you are 100% responsible for your actions. There is no one else to blame. Like Billy Bixbee demonstrated in the opening story, as individuals we can no longer afford to ignore our dragons. We know that what is ignored grows and multiplies. They may have been soft on you up to this point, sending a small lesson or nudge here and there in an attempt to get your attention. But if you keep ignoring the signs, you can feel certain a storm is brewing. A wrath even. Quickly what was once a kitten-sized nudge will grow into dragons that demand you act or face tremendous consequences.

Now is choice time.

Will you Circle Up and choose to ask for help by reaching out to a men's team at Circle Up? Or will you hide out, be the lone wolf, and pull your mask on tightly avoiding the dragons you know you need to face but haven't?

Will you Circle Up and choose your new life, your new discipline, and your success actions, over and over, until the universe happily bends to your will? Or will you allow yourself to be overcome by your addictions and your current personality, remaining bound in a rut of regret and hopelessness?

I know what I would do. What the men engaged in Circle Up are doing. We're not leaving our better futures to chance. We're deciding to make a change. We are choosing fuck it!

You too have that opportunity. We invite you to make your first "fuck it "the decision to reach out to Circle Up and be part of changing your life alongside a group of men who have your back. You're not alone on this journey. We too experience doubt. We too have dragons that need facing. But most importantly, we are facing them, and we are choosing to face them together.

From the moment of that first "fuck it, "you're already becoming less of a man who sits on the couch listening to the voices of doubt and more of a man who boldly steps on to the battlefield. The battlefield is where you learn. This is where you discover your next step. And this is what keeps the voice of doubt at bay. Fear faced may cause injury, but the warrior inside you will live to fight again. This is the way of the superior man.

You are a warrior. You are a man of action. You were born to fight.

Circle Up!

San Marcos, Guatemala - June 2021

CHAPTER SUMMARY:

If you believe there's no such thing as dragons, you're in for a rude awakening. Dragons, that in which we avoid and hide from as men, hold the power to either liberate us, or destroy us. Your dragons are like the weeds in your garden, what you ignore, grows and multiplies. That which you fear, that which you neglect, will come back to bite you more fiercely and with more vigor than ever before. Whatever that dragon represents in your life is your battlefield. This chapter is all about equipping you with the philosophies, the science, and the challenges—your armory—to become the type of warrior who takes action in the face of his doubts and fears.

Resource Summary

Stay close to the resources, quotes, and thinkers you resonated most with in this chapter. Pay attention to what speaks to your heart. If you said to yourself, "I should check that out, "take action immediately.

1. **Mens Weekend - Sterling-institute.com - Justin Sterling**
2. **Rewired - Gaia.com - Joe Dispenza**
3. *Breaking The Habit Of Being Yourself* - **Joe Dispenza**
4. *The Seasons Of Life* - **Jim Rohn**
5. *Think And Grow Rich* - **Napoleon Hill**
6. *Fly Kicks* - **AC Slater (Wax Motif Remix)**
7. *There's No Such Thing as a Dragon* - **Jack Kent**
8. **Slaying The Dragon Within Us - YouTube - Jordan Peterson**
9. *Atomic Habits* - **James Clear**
10. *Profile of a Champion* - **George Zalucki**
11. *Food Rules: An Eater's Manual* - **Michael Pollan**
12. *The Way Of The Superior Man* - **David Deita**

Self Reflection Opportunity

Once complete, move these notes to your phone. This will serve to summarize what you have learned, as well as ensure the resources, quotes, and ideas you personally resonated with most, are available at your fingertips.

Key points to remember (fill in here):

What is one idea from this chapter that will help me "set a better sail" in my own personal philosophy?

CHAPTER SEVEN:

SLAYING DRAGONS

"Unless you change how you are, you'll always have what you've got."

Jim Rohn

THERE ARE NO SHORTCUTS IN THIS BUSINESS

J.R.R. Tolkien's *The Hobbit*, called, "a flawless masterpiece... One of the most influential books of our generation "by The Times, is a textbook for men in search of the ingredients necessary to become a man who can slay dragons. I remember living in Colombia when I first picked up the book. I quickly lost my sense of self and time, shirking all of my responsibilities, just to learn what was to become of Bilbo the Hobbit, Gandalf the Wizard, their band of a dozen Militant dwarves, and their daunting quest; to reclaim their treasure stolen by the terrible dragon Smaug.

After many close encounters with death by trolls, giant spiders and wolves, goblins and more, the adventurers finally reach the beast and accidentally awaken him from his century long dormancy. Smaug flew into a rage, erupting from the mountain in a fiery wrath heading straight for the neighbouring Lake Town. J.R.R. Tolkien sets the imagination on fire with his description, "My armour is like tenfold shields, my teeth are swords, my claws spears, the shock of my tail is a thunderbolt, my wings a hurricane, and my breath death... Roaring, he swept back over the town... Fire leaped from the dragon's jaws... No fireworks you ever imagined equaled the sights that night. "

With rain falling hard on the roof of our Airbnb in Guatape, Colombia , I was in a trance. Lane 8's electronic music floated in and out of my awareness and I could see Iain dancing in the other room through a crack in my door. Wide eyed, I was reading, but, at the same time, I wasn't. My imagination had become so vivid that I had entered the book and was as much part of the scene as Smaug himself.

Suddenly, a warrior appeared. And this story of fiction, that I had begun reading for entertainment, taught me more about what it meant to be a man than any formal schooling ever had. With buildings collapsing, "No one had dared to give battle to him for many an age; nor would they have dared now, if it had not been for the grim-voiced man (Bard was his name), who ran to and fro cheering on the archers and urging the Master to order them to fight to the last arrow. "

Now with flames all around, men abandoning their posts (including the town's Master, who gave up hope and attempted to escape in the confusion and save himself), and Bard drawing back his yew bow to release a final arrow, a small bird with news from Bilbo and his companions interrupted this last shot. "Look for the hollow of the left breast as he flies and turns above you! "the old thrush instructed.

With Smaug's secret weakness revealed, Bard drew back his final arrow, and said "Black arrow! I have saved you for last. You never failed me and always have I recovered you. I had you from my father and he of old. If ever you came from the forges of the true king under the Mountain, go now and speed well! "Holding my breath now, I could see through Bard's eyes as Smaug swooped down again lower than ever exposing his diamond belly that, "glittered white with sparkling fires of gems in the moon-but not in one place. "

Laying on a bed in Colombia, but somehow simultaneously in Middle Earth with Bard, the flames, and the screaming villagers, I became the black arrow. As I sped through the air and pierced the dragon's heart, I said to myself, "What nobody will ever see is the decades of blood, sweat, and tears that made this single shot possible. Bard is the dragon slayer and there are no short-cuts in the business of dragon slaying."

Standing now, I walked to the bathroom and repeated to myself in the mirror, "There are no short-cuts in the business of dragon slaying." I started replaying all of the moments in my life that I cut corners, took the easy way out, and even lied to get ahead. I decided then and there that that isn't the man I want to be. I decided that I wanted to be a warrior with honour and with courage and with commitment. I wanted to be like Bard, a dragon slayer.

You may be thinking to yourself, "Great story, but that's all it is, just a fiction… "to which I relate a powerful idea Iain shares with me frequently from G.K Chesterton, in which he said, "Fairytales say that apples were golden only to refresh the forgotten moment when we found that they were green. They make rivers run with wine only to make us remember, for one wild moment, that they run with water." Acts of heroism and examples of the true warrior, the dragon slayer, exist all around us.

Bard's tale and J.R.R. Tolkien's writing stirred in me the burning desire to remember my roots as a warrior and to consider deeply, "Who is the man I've always wanted to be?"

Now, I ask you the same. Who is the man you've always wanted to be?

And what's the gap between that man and who you're being today? With a vision for your new future and a daily discipline to help you walk the path towards that man, you're well on your way. But becoming this man is a lifelong process. It never ends. This process is also individual. Every man's dragons are different because every man's vision is unique. Earl Nightingale defined success as "the realization of a worthy ideal. "No one gets to decide what your worthy ideal will be. This is your life.

The only person that defines success for you is you. For Bard, that was to be a warrior and serve in the military. For me, it's to become fully self-sufficient as a man and to become a leader in the personal development industry like my hero, Jim Rohn. But, for you, your dragon may be to grow a successful business or to become a professional athlete or to become sober and volunteer in help groups. Your path is unique and it is my hope that this book, like *The Hobbit* did for me, has stirred inside you a desire to become that man.

For that man, and that man only, is capable of slaying the dragons in your life. Right now, you have the choice to live a life of fate or to create your own destiny. With the tools from the last chapter on becoming the type of man who consistently steps onto the battlefield in your life, I offer these final philosophies that, if implemented, can create quantum leaps between who you are now and the man you've always wanted to be.

It's brilliant to *face* your dragons and become a man who takes action in the face of fear. But *slaying* dragons is another chapter of your journey altogether.

Whether it's because you want the vast treasure happily paid to men of mastery, or simply the personal satisfaction of knowing you've become a man of courage, commitment, and honour, the following ideas are the best I've found to help guide you in this noble pursuit. As visionary entrepreneur Marc Castel, one of the men who best role-models the man I've always wanted to be, says, "Go forward with kindness, courage and curiosity. "There's no shortcuts in the business of dragon slaying.

Becoming Fully Self-Sufficient

As men interested in pursuing a worthy ideal and becoming successful, we need to ensure we're strong in more than just our mental health. We need to become fully self-sufficient. Justin Sterling, Founder of the Sterling Institute of Relationships, has been coaching men for more than three decades and says, "If a man doesn't know his purpose today, he should make his purpose to become fully self-sufficient as a man. "The foregoing sentence is worth reading a second time, and a third, and a forth. It's worth reading aloud! It's that important.

What does it mean to be fully self-sufficient? It means that you're able to maintain yourself without outside aid. You need nothing from nobody. This doesn't mean you don't ask for help or are generous to others. It is simply a worthwhile aim for men to become so independent that they can be a pillar of strength for themselves, their brothers, and their community. Self-sufficiency, therefore, clearly extends beyond the parameters of mental health into the world of holistic wellbeing. Wellbeing consists of the collective health of:

1. **Mental health**
2. **Physical health**
3. **Spiritual health**
4. **Emotional health**
5. **Financial health**

Each of these pillars of our life are interconnected and impact the success and health of the others. For example, poor physical health, like my back pain, dramatically reduces my quality of life and affects my mental health. Furthermore, if you're behind on your bills or are in debt, it's highly likely that this financial strain will induce stress, negatively impacting other areas of your well being like your emotional, mental, and physical health.

Imagine Bard woke up that fateful morning and, instead of getting to work soldiering, stayed in bed all day because of debilitating back pain. Or that he had sold his bow a few days earlier because he needed to pay his money lender. Or as we discussed throughout this book, he saw the dragon and instead of stepping up with courage and rallying his men, he became overwhelmed with doubt and fear and fled his people like the Town's cowarding Master. What would have happened?

The village would have been toast. And Smaug would still be hoarding his treasure as dragons do. Without self-sufficient men and women, our communities have no chance at thriving. Again, being self-sufficient doesn't mean that you're living in a silo, it just means you do not *need* anything from anyone. This is powerful. Not needing anything does not mean that you don't ask for and accept help, for there's no such thing as a self-made man. On the contrary, it means that you're emotionally and mentally resilient enough to know when and how to ask for help and to gladly accept it when appropriate.

Simply put, what being self-sufficient means is that you are no longer a boy. You are a man. A man takes 100% responsibility for his life and that is his greatest strength. Jim Rohn believed that this acceptance of personal responsibility is the highest form of human maturity. It is the hallmark of masculinity. For the self-sufficient man, his greatest source of confidence is to know that, without a shadow of a doubt, he is rock solid. The self-sufficient man says, "I know who I am and do not need anything external to satisfy me or make me happy."

Do not misinterpret this concept with the idea of the lone-wolf. The self-sufficient man is the furthest from it. The lone-wolf is severely deficient in his mental and emotional health. He believes that, because he doesn't need anything from anyone, he will take on the challenges of life alone. Fearful of both asking for help as well as being helped. On the other hand, the self-sufficient man believes that because he doesn't *need* anything from anyone, he *can* and *will* include his brothers and community in his life.

He knows that we are stronger together, and, because he is self-sufficient, he is not only of great value to those around him, he has the mental and emotional health to be supported in the advancement of his life and purpose. These are the men that we turn to during a crisis. It is these men who have the strength to serve their families and communities. And it is these men who leave the world better than they found it.

How To Become Self-Sufficient

If you're not fully self-sufficient today, do not let this section discourage you. Few men have taken on and completed this project. I, for one, am the first to admit that I am not fully self-sufficient. But you better believe I'm conscious of it and on the path! Therefore, do not be overly critical if you are not there today.

Our ambition is to become fully self-sufficient, not to have everything figured out at this moment. When you surround yourself with men who have a common purpose, like becoming fully self-sufficient, you will find out that you are not alone and can begin making progress quickly.

An easy formula for becoming self-sufficient is:

In the area of your strengths, generously serve those in need. On the other hand, in the area of your weaknesses, ask for help from those who're strong.

They say it takes a village to raise a child and I agree. Asking for help when you're struggling, and serving others when you're strong, is how a community works. In high school, I struggled desperately with my mental health. If it wasn't for the hands and love of my friends, my family, and community, it's likely that I never would have gathered the necessary strength and desire to improve my life. When I was struggling, those who loved me became pillars of strength for me to lean on.

Moreover, today, as a man who has been working to become wiser for the last decade, I have found strength in my mental, emotional, spiritual, and financial health. However, I am still a work in progress. My dragon to slay is my physical health. And as you know, in this business, there are no short-cuts.

In August of 2021, after rigorous self-reflection, I realized that I wasn't walking my talk. Surprising all of my friends and family, I decided to return back to Canada after nine months of living abroad. At the time, I was surrounded by the best of friends, unlimited opportunity for peak experiences, and living in one of the most beautiful places in the world, Lake Atitlan, Guatemala. But I knew that I wasn't living my purpose. I wasn't fully self-sufficient.

In fact, by that time, my back pain had become a 8/10 and I was suffering. Every day, I had to filter my decisions through a lens of "Would this make it worse? "and began to dread my favourite people asking me to spend time with them. With my quality of life and mental health quickly deteriorating, I decided to pull the trigger and move back home with my parents and sister. What I was doing and how I was living wasn't working. I needed to step back and take James Clear's advice and be intentional about my environment.

The lifestyle of my environment at the time included a lot of dancing and a lot of socializing, amongst other things. All of which, therapeutic for most everyone present, was not helping me heal. At twenty-six years old and after five years of living independently, I had to swallow my pride and make the decision to move back home and lean on my family. This wouldn't have been possible if I didn't have the mental and emotional strength to ask for help. Nor would my family have been able to be there when I needed a pillar of strength, if it were not for their own financial, mental, and emotional self-sufficiency.

The first step to identifying where you can ask for help is to measure the degree to which you're self-sufficient today. I offer you the questions we use at Circle Up in order to help men identify their current strengths and weaknesses.

Self-Reflection Opportunity

Self-Sufficiency

On a scale from 1-5, 5 being the highest, rate yourself. This brief questionnaire will reveal to you the gap between where you are today and becoming fully self-sufficient. Be honest with yourself. Bullshitting yourself may save your feelings in the short-term, but it will only cover up the work to do and set you up for a future disappointment.

Physical Health

1.1 Physical Self Sufficiency - I am reliable to take care of my health—doctors, gyms, etc.

(1 is lowest, 5 is highest)

1 2 3 4 5

1.2 Physical Self Sufficiency - I am proud of my physical condition and maintain it.

(1 is lowest, 5 is highest)

1 2 3 4 5

1.3 Physical Self Sufficiency - If my woman could no longer have sex, I would not have a problem with it.

(1 is lowest, 5 is highest)

1 2 3 4 5

1.4 Physical Self Sufficiency - I reliably keep my home, room and or office clean and usable.

(1 is lowest, 5 is highest)

1 2 3 4 5

Total (4 being lowest, 20 being perfection)

/ 20

Emotional Health

2.1 Emotional Self Sufficiency - It doesn't bother me when others think poorly of my decisions, actions, or self.

(1 is lowest, 5 is highest)

1 2 3 4 5

2.2 Emotional Self Sufficiency - I am rarely overworked and have no problem saying no.

(1 is lowest, 5 is highest)

1 2 3 4 5

2.3 Emotional Self Sufficiency - When criticized or rejected, I am unphased emotionally.

(1 is lowest, 5 is highest)

1 2 3 4 5

2.4 Emotional Self Sufficiency - I immediately take responsibility for my fuckups.

(1 is lowest, 5 is highest)

1 2 3 4 5

Total (4 being lowest, 20 being perfection)

/ 20

Spiritual Health

3.1 Spiritual Self Sufficiency - I find peace and happiness within myself.

(1 is lowest, 5 is highest)

1 2 3 4 5

3.2 Spiritual Self Sufficiency - I don't compare myself or evaluate myself based on my partners or friends happiness.

(1 is lowest, 5 is highest)

1 2 3 4 5

3.3 Spiritual Self Sufficiency - I am clear about the difference/contribution I make in the world and am regularly involved in it.

(1 is lowest, 5 is highest)

1 2 3 4 5

3.4 Spiritual Self Sufficiency - My satisfaction is internally driven, not based on feelings or results.

(1 is lowest, 5 is highest)

1 2 3 4 5

Total (4 being lowest, 20 being perfection)

/ 20

Mental Health

4.1 Mental Self Sufficiency - I can be counted on to make snap decisions when the importance is high.

(1 is lowest, 5 is highest)

1 2 3 4 5

4.2 Mental Self Sufficiency - I rarely doubt the decisions I make.

(1 is lowest, 5 is highest)

1 2 3 4 5

4.3 Mental Self Sufficiency - I prefer to lead rather than to follow.

(1 is lowest, 5 is highest)

1 2 3 4 5

4.4 Mental Self Sufficiency - I can easily get out of my head when I need to take action.

(1 is lowest, 5 is highest)

1 2 3 4 5

Total (4 being lowest, 20 being perfection)

/ 20

Financial Health

5.1 Financial Self Sufficiency - I am regularly ahead of my bills and financial obligations.

(1 is lowest, 5 is highest)

1 2 3 4 5

5.2 Financial Self Sufficiency - I am aware of my net worth and it is growing.

(1 is lowest, 5 is highest)

1 2 3 4 5

5.3 Financial Self Sufficiency - I am not dependent on friends or family for loans or day to day expenses.

(1 is lowest, 5 is highest)

1 2 3 4 5

5.4 Financial Self Sufficiency - My word and what I value take importance over simply making money.

(1 is lowest, 5 is highest)

1 2 3 4 5

Total (4 being lowest, 20 being perfection)

/ 20

Now, add up all of your scores and total them below.

Test Total (20 being lowest, 100 being perfection)

/100

Note: These results are subjective.

Note that if you find these scores harsher than you might consider appropriate, this could mean that you were more self-critical than necessary when completing the questions. Remember these results are subjective based on your own self-report. This can occur if you were feeling temporarily or chronically unhappy or anxious, or were hungry, angry or judgmental when you completed the questions.

What has this exercise brought to your attention about where you are/ where you want to go? (fill in here)

Key Point: Gather strength, but do not dwell.

When we struggle with our mental health, for example, we actively need support from our peers and the world. And that's perfectly fine, *temporarily*. When we're struggling, we should happily accept the support, love, and care of those who want us to do well. We need to take the time to gather strength and energy so that we can come back stronger, creating a cycle of Circling Up and mutual support. This is one of the fundamental purposes of community and our men's teams at Circle Up; we're stronger together.

What we want to avoid here is taking advantage of this help and getting too comfortable. When I moved back home, I made it clear it was temporary. I meant that. One of the first conversations I had with my parents was that I was there to gather strength, not to be their little boy again. "My purpose, "I told them, "is to become fully self-sufficient so that I can again go back out into the world and explore and love and serve. "Therefore, while my time there was rejuvenating and relaxing, it was also disciplined and focused.

So if it takes you a year, two, or five, to gather the necessary strength to take care of yourself again, so be it. But don't dwell here inside of that struggle. Every man needs to know that it's okay to not be okay. And that it's okay to be honest with yourself and others about where you are and what help you need. We've all been there in some way or another. Including myself, as of this writing. Asking for help in these moments is the strongest thing you can do. It is the definition of Circling Up.

But with this awareness, now what? Will you change? Will you do the necessary things in order to improve your life? Or will you continue doing what you've always done, getting the same results you've always got?

It's so important, as we discussed in chapter two, to take off your mask with men you trust so as to feel deeply what you need to feel and soak up all there is to learn about yourself in that pain and suffering. But, know deep down, that you have a choice to move beyond your current circumstances. You have the capacity to heal and the capacity to thrive. And together, we will.

Key Point: Think of your self-sufficiency or lack thereof as a cup with water in it.

The typical self-care approach is to fill up your cup and then pour that water into others. You rest and gather strength, and then you go into the world and try to make a difference. This is not the case with the fully self-sufficient men in my life.

Their capacity is so great, they are such a pillar of strength, that they never pour out of their cup. These men go internal; they focus on loving, respecting, and trusting themselves, becoming fully self-sufficient, and instead of filling up and emptying their cups, they're literally filling themselves up to the point where their cups are running over in abundance. Because of that, all of the lives of those around them are impacted by that spillage.

My dad is an example of one of those men. At seventy-nine years old, he is in better shape than most of the fifty year olds I know. Rather than stopping and starting, you don't stop taking care of yourself. You keep taking care of yourself. You keep loving yourself. You keep living from your heart and your deepest truth. It's from that place where the rest of the world gets to receive your light and your love.

My challenge to you is to do as Justin Sterling proposed: if you do not have a purpose, or you are not fully self-sufficient, *make* your purpose to become fully self-sufficient. It may be one of the most important dragons you slay in your life. Iain, in the way only he can, wrote about dragons in this poem:

Dragon Dreaming

The are not problems,
Only dragons that we
Ourselves create,
For the thrill
And satisfaction
Of slaying.

Yet we may find
To our surprise,
Ourselves bested
By a beast,
That was
Actually only
Preparing us
For the one
Over the Horizon.

And maybe
We weren't
Meant too
Slay it either.

But rather
Ride it
And
Hold the
Reigns
Of fire.

Flying
Wherever
We choose.

Written by Iain Gabriel

So, whether it's because you want to become successful, find a committed relationship, or dig yourself out of the hole you're in, fulfilling this purpose will prepare you to slay, or ride, dragons more than any other accomplishment you can experience in this lifetime. Whatever area of wellbeing you're struggling in, go back and use the exercises outlined in the previous chapter to create a discipline in that facet of your life, and start making progress.

Gather strength, but do not dwell. The world, like with Bard in *The Hobbit*, is counting on it.

Slow Is Smooth And Smooth Is Fast

In the pursuit of self-sufficiency, your first step is to become the type of man who consistently acts in the face of his doubt and fear. By following the steps outlined in the previous chapter, you're already well on your way. Next, as David Deita beautifully advocates in his international bestseller *The Way Of The Superior Man* is to intimately learn your edge and to take action that leans just beyond it.

I have found this practice of learning to lean just beyond your edge the most challenging of all disciplines in the pursuit of becoming the man I've always wanted to be.

Learning your edge requires radical honesty, rigorous self-reflection, patience and humility. David describes your edge as, "Where you stop short, or where you compromise your fullest gift, and instead, cater to your fears. "He expands on this concept by demonstrating that there are two common ways that men "cater "to their fears. First, through laziness, and, secondly, through delusion. After introspection, I see clearly that I have been guilty of both.

Fear And Laziness

In the first bucket, I have been lazy, but mostly fearful, in my relationships with women. Either by letting women who excite me pass me by for fear of rejection, or through spending months too long in relationships that I was no longer happy in. This common error of judgement and personality, as we've explored, is due to doubt. "Your insecurity, "David writes, "causes you to doubt yourself, and so you take the easy way, not even approaching your real edge or real gift. "

Because this cycle of doubt-induced-inaction has been discussed throughout, I'll simply emphasize the importance of continuing to diligently beware of this common shortcoming. These men, including myself in these moments, lack the enthusiasm, depth, and gravitas of a man living at his edge. I know, without a shadow of a doubt, that if you've read this far, you have incredible potential inside of you.

Continue to say "fuck it, "breaking loose from the shackles you placed on yourself with your own doubt, moving beyond that fear, comfort and laziness, into a man who tussles, plays with, and, as David writes, "makes love with the present moment while giving your unique gift. "

Self-Reflection Opportunity: In what areas of your life are you allowing fear or laziness hold you back?

Fear And Delusion

In the second bucket, I have been mostly delusional in my relationship with my physical health. Either by pushing far beyond my capacity and edge, injuring myself in the process, or by believing that I had all of the prerequisite knowledge needed to coach myself through my injuries. Unfortunately, as we explored in chapter one's overview of our current mental health landscape, Einstein pointed out that, "We cannot solve our problems with the same thinking we used when we created them."

Not surprisingly, David believes this common error in judgement is also due to insecurity. He writes, "Your insecurity may lead you to push, push, push, seeking to become victorious over your own sense of lack. "This is a powerful insight into the masculine. When we push far beyond our edge, we demand more than our capacity realistically allows. We stress ourselves unnecessarily. Or, in the case of my physical health, my delusion and naivety lead me to believe I didn't need a weightlifting coach and so I pushed beyond my breaking point.

David helped me realize that my insecurity led me to disrespect my body, a mistake that I am still in the process of learning from and reconciling seven years later. Avoid this common shortcoming. Be honest with yourself about where you're pushing too far beyond your edge. David writes that you can identify this imbalance by paying close attention to where you are "living a false life, off-center, tense, or missing the moment. "You need not injure, disrespect, or delude yourself as I have. Instead learn to be honest by dropping your mask with yourself and your men and meet yourself where you're at before you take yourself where you want to go.

Self-reflection opportunity: In what areas of your life are you being delusional and reaching too far beyond your edge?

Leaning Beyond Your Edge

Fortunately, I have examples of where I've found this sweet spot in my life. Looking to develop my confidence after my depression as a teenager, I joined my parents in their first business venture. In the beginning, I watched them deliver dozens and dozens of sales presentations for the family business, while I sat on the sidelines refusing to participate.

Unable to muster the courage on my own, my dad started asking me to chime in on what I thought as he spoke to prospects. Reluctantly, I shared ideas here and there, even though I thought I was making a fool out of myself. Apparently I didn't completely blow it because, eventually, he had me take on 10% of the presentation while he did the remaining 90%. Over the course of a few months, I grew dramatically. He had me presenting 20%, then 50%, and, eventually, leading the entire meeting. By this point, which was almost a year into being in business, I became the type of man who had no problem presenting my prepared talk. My confidence was skyrocketing.

Never did I reach too far, and never did my environment allow me to become lazy or comfortable. I had found my edge and was leaning just beyond it, over and over.

When I started getting wins under my belt by growing our sales, others started to notice. Again, they helped push me slightly beyond what I would have done on my own and I was now standing in front of a group of three, five and sometimes even ten people to share our business. In less than a year, I went from being the kid who walked into a business meeting wearing sweatpants with palms sweaty, throat dry, and unable to speak up, to being the young man that people wanted to introduce their prospects to. From there, my success expanded.

I did over a hundred sales presentations before I graduated from Georgian College a few years later. This prepared me for when I met the CEO of Fiix Software, Marc Castel, in 2016, so that I could land my dream job, only two days after graduating. At Fiix, I made tens of thousands of sales calls and hundreds of thousands of dollars over four years.

I joined Toastmasters, started my own Club, and over three years accomplished the highest distinction they have to offer, the Distinguished Toastmaster.

I was accepted into Venture For Canada, whose mission is to foster the entrepreneurial skills and mindsets of postsecondary graduates, and once again found myself surrounded by incredible leaders and thinkers.

I began volunteering with Jack.org and sharing my story with my network and, in the last five years, have given over a hundred presentations about mental health.

None of this came quickly, though.

Think of leaning just beyond your edge like getting braces. First, orthodontists assess the status of your teeth today. Then, they create a plan so that the braces shift your teeth ever so slightly over a few years. At first, it's uncomfortable, until it's not. Once the forward progress becomes your new normal, they introduce another slight shift repeating the process of discomfort, followed by adaptation, followed by discomfort, followed by arrival. What was once just a dream, became a set of straight teeth. I used the exact same process to grow my confidence and encourage you to do the same for your vision of the future.

The seeds of these fruits that I now enjoy were all planted at seventeen years old when I walked into my first business meeting wearing sweatpants, unable to make eye-contact with any of my parents' colleagues. I've come so far since my depression in High School that, sometimes, I think that I must have gotten lucky. But when I remember how hard it was in the beginning, and how I just kept putting one foot in front of the other, leaning into my discomfort, I realized that I was simply and unconsciously applying *The Way Of The Superior Man*.

I don't say this to brag, for I think I've made it clear that I am just as much on this path as any other man. I share my successes to reinforce to you, and to myself, that with humility, discipline, and faith, any dream is possible.

Key Point: Success leaves clues.

The importance of leaning just beyond your edge can be communicated in many different ways. Jerzy Gregoryk, for example, the World Olympic Weightlifting Champion and guest on multiple of the world's most popular podcasts like the Tim Ferriss Show, talks about this principle through the idea of micro progression. He says to imagine the person who's broke and then wins the lottery.

What happens to all the money?

Soon enough, it's squandered and they are broke again.

Why is this?

This phenomena happens because, as Jim Rohn said, "If you don't grow out where the money is, it will come back to where you are." Jerzy said the same thing is true for weight loss. If you take a 200lb person and make them 150lbs by snapping your fingers, they will quickly regain all the weight because their brain is still that of a 200lb person. In Jerzy's interview with Tim Ferriss he said that the pursuit of anything *worthwhile* in life takes at least five years. And anything *world class*, at least ten. One of his friends is a Russian Olympic gymnastic coach and agrees, telling him he needed at least ten years to make a National Champion.

Why?

He said it's because, if he doesn't have ten years, he will break the athlete. It takes ten years for the body to adapt and, without it, he would progress too quickly and the athlete would eventually injure himself as I did. "Anyone who wants to do it faster," he said, "will not make it." All of these masters, these world class men, like Jim Rohn, Jerzy Gregorek, Joe Dispensa, James Clear, James Allen, Justin

Sterling, Eric Windeler, David Deita and so many more, seem to be saying the same thing in a different way.

What are all these men trying to communicate to us about self-mastery, the most important dragon to slay of all?

Slow is smooth and smooth is fast. ☯[42]

That the long path is actually the short one. That the slow route is actually the fast route. In other words, learn how to find your edge, then take action just beyond it.

Self Reflection Opportunity:

1. **Count your wins. Where are you leaning just beyond your edge? Where are you, as David Deita says, "owning your fear, and leaning just beyond it?"**

2. **What can you learn from these successes so as to apply to the areas you identified you're either being lazy or delusional?**

    a. **Laziness:**

    b. **Delusion:**

42 ☯ **Philosophy Footnote:** *"Slow is smooth and smooth is fast." - Cole Rowden*

Do not wish to slay dragons out of luck, by chance, or by skipping steps. That's what I did in the gym as a teenager. I'm still paying the price of that insecurity, impatience, and naivety today.

Remember, there are no short-cuts in this business. Bard disciplined himself his whole life for the fateful moment he released his black arrow into Smaug's heart. Instead of wishing and praying that your circumstances would change quicker than it is, choose to be radically honest about your edge and to patiently discipline yourself to lean just beyond it. David believes that very few men have the guts for this practice. Go out into the world and prove him wrong. Constantly. In everything you do.

Where Will You Be In Five Years?

In chapter five, we discussed in great detail the importance of surrounding yourself with men and influences who're intentionally focused on their own personal development. These men are doing the work of making their unconscious conscious, learning to set a better sail, and are improving themselves, their relationships, and taking action on the path of becoming the men they've always wanted to be.

Why did we do that?

We did that because Jim Rohn taught the difference between who you are today and who you will be in five years depends mostly on the books you read and the people you spend the majority of your time with. In *Atomic Habits*, James Clear proved that, by describing your environment as, "the invisible hand that shapes human behavior. "

If there are always cookies in the house and you're trying to lose weight, you're shooting yourself in the foot. If you're trying to stop drinking, but your buddies hit the bar every night, your odds of replacing that addiction are slim to none. In great detail, James demonstrates that while motivation, talent, and effort are important, "the surprising thing is, especially over a long time period, your personal characteristics tend to get overpowered by your environment. "

Therefore, if we assume this philosophy is true (and I have found it true for myself time and time again), the easiest and most reliable way to ensure we arrive where we want to arrive in five years is to be intentional about who we spend our time with.

Pay Attention To Your Direction

Personally, I met my best friend Iain when I was eighteen. As you now know, at the time, I was seriously lacking in confidence and belief in myself. Since then, as a result of all of our time spent as roommates, business partners, work colleagues, and best friends travelling around the world, I've grown dramatically in the areas of Iain's strengths; my creativity, confidence, and even my sense of humour. In *Atomic Habits,* James points out that this proximity has a powerful effect on our behaviour.

Jim Rohn would agree as he is responsible for popularizing the idea that, "You become the average of the five people you spend the most time with. "So we tend to pick up the habits, mannerisms, and even the inside jokes of the people around us. The closer we are to someone, the more likely we are to be like them. This is why it's critical to have a vision for your future.

If you know where you want to go, then you can intentionally choose which relationships and communities align with that new vision. Without direction, on the other hand, it doesn't matter who you hang out with. By not knowing where you're going, you won't know which associations are having a positive or negative influence on your life. It's only when you're clear about your direction that you can set up your environment to work for you, instead of against you.

Fortunately, we've laid all of this groundwork already. If you've been an active participant throughout this book, you've done the work of identifying your addictions, your commitments, and your vision for the future. If you haven't, I invite you to go back to get the most out of this book and our time together. While there is tremendous value in reading alone, I encourage you to go beyond "going through the motions" and, instead, finish what you started.

By reading this book, you're planting the seeds of these ideas and philosophies into the fertile soil that is your mind. By completing the exercises, however, you're like the farmer who diligently waters and takes care of his crop all summer. Nothing can replace this effort. And the difference in your harvest come fall could be the difference between "just another book "and a moment in time when your whole life changed. That potential is in your effort and how you choose to look at these exercises.

PAY ATTENTION TO YOUR ASSOCIATIONS

The most effective approach you can take today to thoughtfully design your environment is by choosing, as James Clear suggests, "a culture where your desired behaviours are the normal behaviour of the group. "For example, when I wanted to improve my public speaking skills, I joined a Toastmasters club. When I wanted to become a better dancer, I started taking salsa lessons.

In both cases, I first knew where I wanted to go, and then, aligned my environment with that intention so as to pull me towards my desired future. Public speaking skills and confidence on the dance floor were normal ways of being for these communities and so, by investing my time with them, I improved my skills naturally, without struggle, simply through association.

Now, this doesn't mean there was no discomfort. You can count on discomfort, fear, and doubt to arise when you're surrounded by individuals with skills and character you want to embody. This is a gift. "Fear needs to become your friend, "David Deita said in *The Way Of The Superior Man*. Be *with* the fear. Being with the fear and staying at your edge, allows real transformation to occur.

Someone once said that if you're the smartest person in any given room, you're probably in the wrong room. Commit to surrounding yourself with disciplined, skilled, and highly intelligent individuals who align in the direction of your new life. You will find that they pull you there faster than you could have ever imagined.

It worked for me. In my confidence by participating in my parents first business, for my communication skills from my weekly Toastmasters attendance, and in my creativity, openness to experience, and my wonder and love for life because of my friendship with Iain. You too are only one relationship, or one community, away from personal transformation. Who knows which new expanded association will make the difference in making the next five years of your life the best five years of your life.

Self-Reflection Opportunity

Jim Rohn categorizes associations into three groups: expanded associations, limited associations, and dissociations. If you're ready to make quantum leaps in your life, choosing to spend more time with expanded associations, the people you want to emulate, and less or no time with limited and dissociations, is how you bring forth the vision for your new future.

1. **Identifying Expanded Associations**

Based on your direction, consider what group or community you could join that would put you in the best position to change your personal reality. If you're looking to get sober, you could join Alcoholics Anonymous. If you're looking to make more money, you could join a mastermind with high income earners. Or if you're like I was, asking the types of questions that made this book possible, like "How to be honest about your personal struggles? What does empowered masculinity look like? "Or "How do I get out of my head and into action? " we invite you to consider making Circle Up part of your journey.

My example

Intention: I am grateful for my relaxed, strong, and playful mind, body and spirit.

Communities and places where these types of people likely meet:

1. Weightlifting teams, like a powerlifting or olympic weightlifting gyms
2. Spiritual communities where they practice meditation, yoga, and mindfulness, like Eagles Nest in San Marcos, Guatemala, or an equivalent community depending on where I'm living
3. Dance studios where I can learn latin, ecstatic, or contact dances

YOUR TURN

Intention:

Communities and places where these types of people likely meet:

1.
2.
3.

2. Commit To Spending Time With Them

A recommendation I love and have used ever since reading Tim Ferriss's New York Times bestselling book *Four Hour Workweek* is to set a three-step action plan. One you can do right now, the second you can do within twenty-four hours, and a third action you will take within the next week. I highly recommend using this simple three-step action plan any time you want to immediately get yourself our of doubt and into "fuck it."

MY EXAMPLE

Next steps:

1. Right now – I will commit to calling Ryan (a good friend and owner of Keep Growing Fitness, who has a powerful track record for helping individuals recover from sport injuries) that I want an appointment with him this week

2. Within the next twenty-four hours – I will go for a walk and listen to the one-hour podcast with Aubrey Marcus, Founder of Onnit, and Olympic Weightlifting Champion and Co-Creator of The Happy Body exercise program, Jerzy Gregorek

3. Within the next seven days – I will complete my assessment with Ryan and talk to him about the next appropriate actions

YOUR TURN

Next Steps:

1. **Right now -**

2. **Within the next twenty-four hours -**

3. **Within the next seven days -**

No need to overthink this. Stop reading now and complete the first action. Now that this action has been taken, you're already on the battlefield. Congratulations! Before reading further, make sure that steps two and three are easy for you to accomplish in the next week. If you continue to keep it simple by taking one step after another, the universe will have no choice but to bend to your will. As a matter of fact, with your first action already taken, it already is.

Key Point: You don't need to cut your current friends out of your life.

Or maybe you do.

Again, expanded associations are anyone that aligns with the direction of your vision for the future. Spending as much time with these people as possible creates a sort of cosmic vortex, pulling the dreams out of your head and making them a reality. "Limited associations, "as Jim puts it, "are the people who aren't necessarily negative influences on you, but they're also not moving you closer to your new personality. " And finally, dissociations are people who are actively pulling you in the direction of a life you've decided is no longer congruent with how you want to think, feel, and act.

Jim said that there are some people you can spend a few days with, but not a few years. Others, a few hours, but not a few days. And some who make you feel drained just by being in their presence. Finding men like my boy Iain can act like a North Star. Iain is an expanded association that brings energy, colour, and enlightenment to my days. After spending virtually *every* day together from 2018-2021, we started a podcast on Spotify called *Till The End* to ensure, no matter how far apart life takes us, we'd have a reason to be connected. When you find men like Iain, when you find brotherhood, you don't let that go.

So, while you may consider letting some of your current friends go, what I've found personally more empowering than focusing on dissociation is to simply spend as much time as possible with the expanded associations and communities that bring you energy and pull you towards your new life. This way, instead of calling a friend and saying, "Hey, Jonathan said you're holding me back, so we can be friends anymore... "you will naturally find yourself wanting to spend more time with people that demonstrate the qualities of character you desire to embody, and have the skills you want to learn.

Most importantly, one of the major focuses of the code of honour we observe in Circle Up is to "Embrace all men. "Spend no time blaming others for where you've arrived today. Instead, starting now, focus exclusively on who you want to be and where you want to go. Then, become it. The man you become will act like a magnetic force whose presence and clarity of vision has the potential to move the men around you from doubt into action. Becoming the man you've always wanted to be is your most selfless contribution to the world. Your light is a bright torch from which the rest of humanity gathers strength.

CIRCLE UP

After a year of struggle and strife working on this book, I mentioned to Iain that I was thinking about hiring a coach. At the time, I had just gotten out of the hospital; I spent two days unable to walk for being an idiot (doing a flip off a 30-foot cliff jump into water) and realized that I needed to change. For hours, painkillers coursing through my veins, I reflected on Morpheus' words in one of my favourite movies of all time *The Matrix*, when he said, "Neo, sooner or later you're going to realize just as I did that there's a difference between knowing the path and walking the path. "The reason the book wasn't complete yet was because I knew the path, but I wasn't walking it.

I told him it was going to be a significant investment, to which, after no hesitation, he replied, "Listen to this, "passing me his headphones. He then played Russ' song "Money on Me. "In only a few minutes, it was clear what he was communicating. Iain took the headphones back and repeated one of Russ' standout lyrics, "I bet on myself and I don't even gamble. "And then, immediately suggested that I send the money to Blake Fly, a man I respect and admire; a man who has already walked down the path I knew only intellectually.

He reminded me that Jim always used to say, "The best investment you can make is one in yourself "and repeated with a grin what we'd just heard from Russ, "betting on yourself isn't a gamble, bro." That night, when I went home, I thought about my experience laying in that Guatemalan hospital bed, painkillers in full effect, going over my life. I knew I had experienced a lot of adventure and excitement in the last year, but I also knew that I had been living in fear. Like every warrior, I experienced a lot of doubt.

I thought about how many times I let my fears keep me off the battlefield. I was violating the exact same philosophy that I so passionately advocated. I realized I was afraid of judgement. Judgement for my body, for my book, and for new beginnings. I realized that I would never become my new self if I couldn't let go of my old self. In order for me to change my personal reality, I knew I needed to make a decision to change my current personality.

That day, I sent the money to Blake Fly. It was the best money I'd ever spent. It was also the moment where, like Bard, releasing his final arrow into Smaug's heart, I slayed my own inner-dragon. The moment I clicked "send "on the money, there was no longer a question of if the book was happening, it had already happened. That decision taught me that every bet you place on yourself is a decision to alter the course of your own personal history.

In HG Wells' *A Short History of the World*, he tells the story of Julius Caesar's defining moment. When his generals told him they'd gone far beyond acceptable boundaries and that he was to bring the army back, he looked them in the eyes and said, "The die is cast. "That decision forever altered history and demonstrates the power of a single "fuck it ". The day that I paid Blake was my cast of the die, another "fuck it, "and the day I shed my old skin. Investing that money was the act of faith that shaped my attitude, my commitment, and the actions and that ultimately led to you reading these words.

The man you've always wanted to be is laying dormant inside of you. All you have to do is get out of the way.

How does one do that?

You do that by betting on yourself and realizing it's not a gamble. Every investment you make in yourself isn't money that disappears, it's money that recycles and multiplies. When you finally say, "fuck it, "and make the decision to invest in yourself, an immediate shift will occur inside of you, as it did for me, from scarcity to abundance.

In Eckhart Tolle's bestselling book *The Power of Now*, he teaches that any action taken from scarcity can only lead to more scarcity. If you hold onto your money with the mindset that it is a scarce resource, it will become one in your life. The same goes for your energy and your love. The fastest way to get love is to give it. The fastest way to get energy is to move. And the fastest way to become more, is to invest in yourself. If you can make a decision to do that, you will be making quantum leaps in becoming the type of man who slays dragons.

Set this happening in motion today. Make the decision to cast your own die, or release your own arrow into the heart of the dragon holding you back, by investing in a men's team with Circle Up or by buying one of the books you resonated most from this one. Trust yourself. Bet on yourself. Walk the path. And most importantly, never shortcut or short change yourself. Distant lands, epic adventures, and treasure hoarding dragons await!

Circle Up!

Toronto, Canada - August 2021

CHAPTER SUMMARY:

It's brilliant to *face* your dragons and become a man who takes action in the face of fear. But *slaying* dragons is another chapter of your journey altogether. Like the oak that sleeps in the acorn, the bird that waits in the egg, the man you've always wanted to be is awaiting your call. The path to this man, the man who is fully self-sufficient, the man of courage and of commitment, the man of honour, has no shortcuts. This chapter is about igniting inside of you the desire to go out into the world and become that man. Few men have the guts for this practice. If it took you 10, 20, or 50 years to become that man, would it be worth it?

Resource Summary

Stay close to the resources, quotes, and thinkers you resonated most with in this chapter. Pay attention to what speaks to your heart. If you said to yourself, "I should check that out, "take action immediately.

1. *The Hobbit* - **J.R.R. Tolkien**
2. *Heretics* - **G. K. Chesterton**
3. **The Strangest Secret - YouTube - Earl Nightingale**
4. **Men's Weekend - Sterling-institute.com - Justin Sterling**
5. *Atomic Habits* - **James Clear**
6. *Way Of The Superior Man* - **David Deita**
7. **Find A Club - Google.com - Toastmasters International**
8. **Become A Jack Talks Speaker - Jack.org**
9. **Careers - Fiix Software**
10. *Till The End - Spotify - Iain Gabriel and Jonathan Andrews*
11. *Money On Me* - **Russ**
12. **Top College Motivational Speaker - Blake Fly**
13. *A Short History of the World* - **H. G. Wells**
14. *Power Of Now* - **Eckhart Tolle**

Self-Reflection Opportunity

Once complete, move these notes to your phone. This will serve to summarize what you have learned, as well as ensure the resources, quotes, and ideas you personally resonated with most, are available at your fingertips.

Key points to remember (fill in here):

What is one idea from this chapter that will help me "set a better sail" in my own personal philosophy?

NOT A CONCLUSION

"Once you realize you don't *have* to do anything, you *can* do anything."

Iain Gabriel

TILL THE END

New York Times bestselling author Tucker Max says that the best books communicate what's on everyone's mind, but no one wants to say. I feel that I have done that here to the best of my current abilities. He also says that the best conclusions don't introduce new information. But we can ignore that advice. This is not the conclusion of Circle Up, this is just the beginning.

The fundamental focus of the philosophy outlined in this book was honesty. Honesty of the thoughts, beliefs, and unconscious conditioning that have shaped your perspective of mental health and masculinity. Honesty about the arrows, traumas, and dragons that have become barriers on your path to living a fully expressed and purposeful life. And honesty about the essential, and likely uncomfortable, steps to be taken if you are to dissolve those barriers and walk the path of becoming the man you've always wanted to be.

Those ideas are outlined here now as chapter summaries. Following these summaries is a final fundamental honesty that I believe is absolutely necessary for anything that's come before it to work.

PART ONE
MAKING THE UNCONSCIOUS, CONSCIOUS

CHAPTER ONE page 19

WHY MEN STRUGGLE WITH MENTAL HEALTH

Mental health struggles are like the fruit the farmer harvests in the fall. The fruit is a symptom. An outcome. The fruit, just like our struggle, is not the root. It is not the seed. When we look at the fruit that is the state of our men's mental health, 75% of suicides are men, every minute a man dies by suicide, and suicide is the #1 health related cause of death between 15-24. We must ask ourselves, "What is the root? Why is there so much struggle? "The answer to which is found in the quality of our thinking. The root of our men's mental health crisis stems from our beliefs and our perceptions about ourselves, masculinity and the world around us. You are not alone.

CHAPTER TWO page 37

HOW MEN GET AWAY WITH MENTAL HEALTH STRUGGLE

Men struggle desperately with addiction, mental health, and suicide, often without even their closest friends and family knowing before it's too late. How is that? It's because we tell you we're fine, but we're lying—we just don't want you to worry. We take all our feelings and hide them because we don't want anyone to hurt us. As warriors, we wear masks. But as warriors who use masks for protection and success, we need to learn where and with whom it's safe to take them off before it's too late.

CHAPTER THREE page 53

WHAT TO DO ABOUT THE MEN'S MENTAL HEALTH CRISIS

Up to this point, our men have been conditioned to struggle alone, hide their pain, and man up. This is not the way. If we continue to perpetuate this level of thinking, we can only create more of the same results. So, how do we create new possibilities for our men, their families, and our communities? A new future requires a new vision. For our men to thrive, we need to stop thinking man up and start thinking Circle Up. Once we personally become the type of men who change our thinking from "man up "to "Circle Up "and from "struggling makes you weak "to "you know I got you, "we give every man in our lives the permission to do the same. Planting new seeds will create a radically new harvest.

CHAPTER FOUR page 73

SELF-CARE: AN ACT OF SELFLESSNESS

The Chinese character for 'man' is fundamentally two sticks leaning against each other. It's this interconnectedness that exposes the importance of learning to effectively take care of ourselves. If 'man' is two sticks leaning against each other, and you're not a stick, but a floppy noodle, how can you be there to help another man? No sports team would ever go into battle without a strategy, yet we run onto the battlefield of our lives every day without a plan for the inevitable adversites, struggles, and even crises we face. Prepare yourself to be strong in the face of life's challenges by developing your own unique mental health action plan. Taking care of yourself is your greatest contribution to the world.

CHAPTER FIVE page 101

MASCULINE CARE: A MENTAL HEALTH REVOLUTION

Masculine care is about finding the fine line between ruthlessness and compassion. All compassion with no ruthlessness and we have our warriors walking around life without ever confronting their injuries and arrows from battle. All ruthlessness with no compassion, and we're perpetuating toxic masculinity conditioning. Neither of these approaches work in the case of men's mental health. One is all heart and no backbone. The other, all spine and no love. Ruthless compassion facilitates masculine relationships so that the action that matters most, normalizing help seeking behaviour during a mental health struggle, is the easiest action to take.

PART TWO
THE FUTURE OF "MAN UP"

CHAPTER SIX page 129

OFF THE COUCH AND ONTO THE BATTLEFIELD

If you believe there's no such thing as dragons, you're in for a rude awakening. Dragons, that in which we avoid and hide from as men, hold the power to either liberate us, or destroy us. Your dragons are like the weeds in your garden, what you ignore, grows and multiplies. That which you fear, that which you neglect, will come back to bite you more fiercely and with more vigor than ever before. Whatever that dragon represents in your life is your battlefield. Equip yourself with the philosophies, the science, and the challenges—your armory—to become the type of warrior who takes action in the face of his doubts and fears.

CHAPTER SEVEN page 171

SLAYING DRAGONS

It's brilliant to *face* your dragons and become a man who takes action in the face of fear. But *slaying* dragons is another chapter of your journey altogether. Like the oak that sleeps in the acorn, the bird that waits in the egg, the man you've always wanted to be is awaiting your call. The path to this man, the man who is fully self-sufficient, the man of courage and of commitment, the man of honour, has no shortcuts. Ignite inside of you the desire to go out into the world and become that man. Few men have the guts for this practice. If it took you 10, 20, or 50years to become that man, would it be worth it?

THE FUTURE IS NOW

The final fundamental honesty required for this philosophy to work is gratitude. In the personal development industry, we get so caught up in the "hustle porn "culture of exceptionalism, and always being and doing more, that we forget the present moment. We forget to be grateful for that in which we already have. We put so much pressure on ourselves to do and accomplish that we forget we're all just figuring it out. I did my best in this book to share authentically and with authority. But this book is not *proof* of having figured anything out. On the contrary, it was the documentation and advocacy of this philosophy that *is* me figuring it out.

It was inside the literal hundreds of hours of writing that I became more conscious of my own dragons, my self-sabotage, and my addictions. I am in no way perfect at following the principles outlined in this book, I am simply on the path of figuring my shit out as anyone else is. The reason this isn't a conclusion is because, well, I'm not sure there is an arrival. Is there really an end to learning? Some point and time when will I have it all figured out? To me, it seems both more likely, and more practical, to think that I will be learning and figuring it out as I go, Till The End.

Isn't that liberating?

We don't have to have it all figured out! It's like taking a leap off the side of a cliff and having faith that you will grow the wings needed to fly as you fall.

From this vantage point, you can pause and take a deep breath. You can drop a lot of the unnecessary pressure you're putting on yourself by having an expectation of where you should be and what you should have accomplished by now. And you can stop rushing around and forcing life. Bob Marley said, "The day you stop racing is the day you win the race. "Without this idea, you wouldn't be holding this book. Realizing that I am doing my best and "just figuring it out," took the pressure off needing to look or sound perfect and gave me the confidence to accept myself fully in this moment. I encourage you to do the same.

To find this balance is to find the middle way. It is as Jim Rohn puts it, "To learn how to be happy with what you have while you pursue all that you want. "For most of my experience, and I believe for most people, we don't approach life this way. At some point, we were conditioned to put off our happiness and enjoyment to some faraway land we may or may not reach. We keep moving the goal post, as Iain consistently points out to me; when I graduate school, I will be happy and grateful, when I get a good job, I will enjoy myself, or when I lose 5olbs, I will be ready to live and love. Unfortunately, this mental rigidity, this pushing off of happiness and a refusal to accept the present moment, is actually the source of our suffering.

Iain reminds me that if you can't enjoy *this* moment now, then you will not enjoy *that* moment then. How true. This experience of unease, anxiety, tension, stress, and worry (too much future), or of guilt, regret, resentment, grievances, sadness, bitterness (too much past), is due to what Eckart Tolle suggests in *The Power of Now:* a lack of present moment awareness, a lack of consciousness. Being present is where gratitude arises. Fortunately, I am extremely optimistic for my life, the brothers I have surrounded myself with in Circle Up, and for the world. Our understanding of the mind, and how to change it, has never looked more promising. This note of optimism is how we part ways.

One of the most exciting developments globally for mental health research is Psychedelic Assisted Psychotherapy. Only today, after decades of suppression, are these psychedelic compounds resurfacing and being acknowledged for their vast potential to help those suffering from too much past or too much future. Michael Pollen describes in his book *How To Change Your Mind* that this lack of presence is likely the symptom of a brain that has become excessively rigid or fixed in its pathways and linkages.

The suffering we experience due to obsessive self-reflection, and an inability to disrupt the deepening grooves of negative thinking, is common in people experiencing depression, anxiety, trauma, and addiction. These people, as his journalism has shown, depicted their depression as a state of disconnection, "feeling separate from other people, their earlier selves, their senses and feelings, their core beliefs and spiritual values, or nature. "Several patients referred to this as feeling like they were living in a mental prison. Others felt stuck in endless circles of destructive rumination, likened to mental gridlock. This was precisely my experience as a teenager.

How can we live in the moment if we're stuck in the mental prison of past and future? How can we be honest about our struggles when we feel separated from the world? We can; only when we change our minds. A healthy brain, as Michael demonstrated, is one that is flexible and supple. This brain feels connected to purpose, people, and nature. And this brain can be built. The world's leading authorities on mental health are testing the potential for Psychedelic Assisted Psychotherapy to heal these challenges of mental rigidity, obsessive and destructive rumination, and disconnection. We are early in our findings (hence not a conclusion), but the potential has researchers, regulators, and much of the mental health community, including me, feeling hopeful.

I'm bullish that just like the Psychedelic Assisted Psychotherapy being conducted in Canadian companies like TheraPsil, and around the world, Circle Up is the future of men's mental health. Michael describes the mystical experience occasioned by psychedelics in the exact same way that we talk about our philosophy at Circle Up; they both have the power to "shake the snow globe "of the mind, disrupting unhealthy patterns of thought, dissolving the ego and sense of separateness from other men and the world, and creating a space of flexibility where new narratives have an opportunity to arise as the snow slowly resettles. This rewiring of the way you think, feel, and act on your mental health and masculinity from "man up "to Circle Up is our mission. It's why we exist.

Both psychedelics and Circle Up sponsor connection and unity, not separation and segregation. Honouring the truth and facing dragons, rather than masks and hiding out. And most importantly, we're committed to—as Psilocybin mushrooms have inspired me and all of the brothers and sisters I have had the honour of sharing their magic with—love, gratitude, and a feeling that no matter what, you know I got you. This is the future of mental health. This future is happening now.

Circle Up

In a world that has never been and felt more separated, Circle Up is a movement of men who are coming together to leave the world better than we found it. While I am bold that our philosophy and Men's Circle is part of a better future for all men, their families, and our communities, I can't quite boast that this book is as powerful as a psychedelic trip. What I can do, in the absence of the compound itself, is send you off with the most beautiful piece of art I have ever found. In my eyes, it creates the same impact of "shaking the snow globe "of any feelings of separateness from other men, or from the world. It will take you on a trip; and depending on the way you look at it, it could change your mind.

Beautiful Tragedy

We are all going to die,
All of these sounds, memories, connections, feelings
will all fade,
ultimately crushed, ruined, obliterated, into an abyss of nothingness never to be seen again.

Like a single rock thrown into the water, never to be considered again.

There was eternity before the throw, eternity after,
and only by chance
did the rock get to be thrown at all.

The time the rock moves through the air and drops in the water is but an instant.

That's all the time there really is.

So how best to spend that time?

The answer to that question
is best answered on a foundation
of understanding the finite nature of that time,
and to create from that,
an urgency to do the things
you would desperately do
before the rock crashes and splashes
into eternal nothingness.

How do you do that without fear and impending doom?

Well, first off, get that at the beginning,
and you make sure that it's real,
because when you truly understand,
when you truly conceptualize that there is a finite time
left available to you,
it should instantly click,
that stress, worry, and overthinking
would be to waste and squander that time.

It's like having the epiphany
that the plane you're on can't land.
The doors are sealed.
There's no escape.
Surely, you will cry when you first find this out,
but then, not despite this realization,
but in-spite of this realization,
you will laugh and dance,
with all your body can muster,
with the people around you,
in this bitter sweet embrace,
this love,
until impending destruction comes,
and overwhelms it all.

It's this sense of ending, which unites us towards common aims.
If life were to go on forever
there would be no urgency.
It's this urgency that we share.
It's this urgency that creates meaning.
It's this urgency that says:
I know that all of this is going to end soon. But I want to share
part of this finite time,
that I have left,
with you.

Written by: Iain Gabriel

If that doesn't shake the snowglobe, I don't know what will.

To a lot of people, talking about death is taboo. ☯[43] But, for a lot of people, so is talking about mental health and suicide. We would rather ignore it, do everything we can to avoid it, and pretend it's not true. Who wants to think about death? So, like we always do at Circle Up, we're facing this dragon. What if instead of being scared and unwilling to embrace this truth we did the opposite? What if reflecting and meditating on that fact was a simple key to living life to the fullest?

---

43 ☯ **Philosophy Footnote:** *Memento Mori is a term in Stoic philosophy to remember our own mortality.*

As Iain pointed out, everyone that I once loved, including myself, will be dead. My parents will die. My closest friends will die. And I know this because some of those I've loved, more than any words could ever describe, are already dead.

You could look at this as morbid, or you can consider, as this book has attempted to reason, that how we see the world is simply a matter of perspective. Surrendering to the truth that everyone I've ever met will eventually die has allowed me to live more fully. Thinking of death is the same as thinking of depression; it brings with it the opportunity for humility, tolerance, open mindedness, and connection. "Meditating on your mortality "as Ryan Holiday from the Daily Stoic suggests, "is only depressing if you miss the point. It is in fact a tool to create priority and meaning. It's a tool that generations have used to create real perspective and urgency. To treat our time as a gift and not waste it on the trivial and vain. Death doesn't make life pointless, but, rather, purposeful. "

Like any dragon in our lives, our mortality can either be our greatest source of suffering, or can carry us across to the next opening. The next expansion. The same taboos and stigmas; depression, mental health, and death, that caused separation in the generation of men before us are the exact same ideas that will unite this one. By moving towards rather than trying to flee this truth that is our sense of ending, we can, as Iain has described, unite in our common aim to make the most of the finite time we have left together.

The philosophy of reconditioning the awareness of death is beautifully woven by my old friend, visionary Canadian tech entrepreneur Mark Castel, when he wrote:

"Because life and our lives are so rare and precious it compels me not to waste them... The universe has conspired to bring us to this amazing Earth, to this unique moment in time. This may be our only opportunity to live, our only opportunity to make a difference. So make your time here matter. Celebrate this gift of life by not wasting it."

How do we live so as to not waste this life?

We don't take ourselves too seriously. We express gratitude for what we do have. We meet ourselves wherever we are today and then take action from there. And finally, we do as Iain suggests, we laugh, we dance, and we love each other. This embrace, after all, is the purpose of Circle Up. It's the purpose of life. So, before passing on to the next chapter in your life, allow Iain's words, as well as Circle Up's mission, to kindle anew in your mind the fire of hope, faith, courage, and tolerance. If you have these states of mind, and a working knowledge of the principles described in this book, all else that you need will come to you when you are ready for it.

Circle Up because every man has mental health and no man struggles alone. Circle Up because no matter the arrows, the suffering, or the dragon, we have the strength to face it. And Circle Up because the men we loved and lost would have wanted us to. Because of them, and their legacy, we have decided that the best way to spend the time we have left in this bitter sweet embrace, this love, is together.

You are not alone.

You can be honest with yourself and your men.

Count your blessings, brother, because you know we got you, till the end.

Circle Up!

Toronto, Canada - August 2021

ACKNOWLEDGEMENTS

Thank you to Jim Rohn, who taught, "Don't wish things were easier, wish you were better." Because of you and your no bullshit take on the importance of personal development, I exposed myself to the world. Like you suggested, I went to the seminars, I watched the movies, I listened to the songs, I read the books, and I allowed life to touch me. You set me on the path to see all that I can do and all that I could become. Every community I've been a part of in the last decade, and that I express gratitude for here, is a result of your influence on my life. Rest In Peace, Jim.

It's been said that you grow into the conversations people have about you and around you. That couldn't be more true than for the family I gained during my parents first business venture as network marketers at All Communications Network (ACN). To Betty-Ann Ellis, Patrick Anderson, David Holland, and hundreds more beautiful souls who took me under their wing at that vulnerable and insecure time in my life, thank you. You all made me believe, once again, that I had something of value to offer the world. You saw in me what I did not see in myself and that has made all the difference.

In 2013, when virtually all of my friends and peers were venturing off to Universities across Canada, I took a year off. I needed time. I wasn't ready to be independent. I wasn't ready to decide what I wanted to do with my life. And I wasn't ready to go into massive debt as a young person struggling with his mental health. Thanks to the encouragement of my sister, Tara, I attended Georgian College with her the next year and found the Henry Bernick Entrepreneurship Center. To my teachers, the leaders at Henry Bernick, and to all the friends I shared major wins with at Georgian, thank you for stretching me just enough outside of my comfort zone to grow without pushing too hard that I landed back onto my parents couch. Those two years instilled in me the confidence needed to venture out on my own and move to the city of Toronto.

From there, I met Marc Castel, James Novak, Shane Skiffington, Daryl Sedgman, Dan Shaw, and all of the leaders and friends that are responsible for helping build Fiix Software into the heart centered company it became. Jim Rohn always said, "Don't ask what you're getting paid here, ask who you're becoming here." I can honestly say, in my four years at Fiix, I did much more than make money; I grew as a man and a leader. Thank you. I know Jim would be proud.

Jim also said, "Work harder on yourself than you do on your job. If you work hard on your job, you can make a living. But if you work hard on yourself, you can make a fortune." In those four years I lived in the city of Toronto, I found Toastmasters, Speaker Slam, Landmark International, Venture for Canada, the Sterling Institute of Relationships and Jack.org. Every one of these communities has helped challenge my thinking, my integrity, and my commitment to personal development. Most importantly, they introduced me to hundreds of brothers, sisters, and mentors who've made an impact in my life through our connection. Y'all know who you are. Thank you for shining your light into my life.

To my men's team, The Foundation, you revealed to me through ruthless compassion that I'm a jerk, that I'm full of shit, and that I am loved by men. Thank you for always having my back.

To the men of the Brotherhood, and to the leaders who blew wind into Circle Up's sails, you're leaving the world better than you found it. Thank you for teaching me how to put my commitment before my ego and for living your men's weekend. None of this is possible without your commitment, passion, and influence.

To my brothers who grabbed their balls and said "Fuck it!" in trusting in our leadership at Circle Up and participating as a founding member, or in one of our men's teams, I am so grateful to be part of your personal development journey. Doing the work of discovering and dissolving the barriers holding you back from becoming the man you've always wanted to be, and then walking that path, requires radical honesty, faith, and disciplined action. You are fucking badasses. In my eyes, you men are the future of empowered masculinity and of men's mental health advocacy.

Writing a book has been a dream of mine for as long as Jim Rohn has been a hero. Tabitha Rose and the team at Life To Paper Publishing make dreams come true. Their professionalism, bravery, and commitment to making an impact on the world through storytelling, inspired me to give my best day in and day out. When I wanted to quit, and I thought about it many times, it was their faith in me, and their belief in our mission at Circle Up, that gave me the strength to finish what I started. Thank you for holding me to a higher standard in my life and in my life's work. #DreamTeam!

To Chad Lennon, aka Pascal Satori aka Grandma Gabriel aka Angel Gabriel aka my attorney and personal philosopher, Iain Gabriel: my brother, my brother, my friend, my friend, my admiration for you has no end. Easily, over one thousand one hundred and eleven times you've said, "Once you realize you don't have to do anything, you can do anything. But you can't do everything, so what will you do?" To that I say, I want to spend part of this finite time that I have left with you, brother. No one has had my back like you. And I know that the last seven years of friendship is just the beginning of our lifelong and likely infinitely longer world tour. You are the boldest, bravest, and highest potential man I've ever met. Whatever the dream, however big the mission (or spliff), I'll be there by your side ready to take it on. My brother, my brother, my friend, my friend, until the last breath, un - 'Till The End.

And finally, to my big brother, Adam, thank you for being a fighter, for your resilience, and for always being one of my most important role models in life. More hockey telepathy in our future soon! To my big sister, Tara, you inspire me with your determination and your strength - it's not cool that you can kick my ass! If life ever gave me a guardian angel, it is you. To my mom, Laura, thank you for never putting unnecessary pressure on me to be something I am not. Instead, your unconditional love and unwavering support, no matter my pursuit, has allowed me to take unconventional routes. We are forever connected. I love you. And to my dad, John, who showed up for me, not just with his words, but with his actions. You showed me that I am not alone. You saved my life. It's because of your love that I know that it only takes one person who cares enough to change the world.

BIBLIOGRAPHY

1. Allen, James. *As A Man Thinketh*. Simon & Schuster. 1903.
2. Andrews, Jonathan. *Circle Up Podcast*. n.d.
3. Andrews, Jonathan, et al. *Till The End*. Podcast. 2021.
4. Ash. *Beausoleil.* Beausoleil. 2019.
5. Assaf. *Lost Souls - AVIRA Remix.* Armada Music. 2020.
6. Beatles, The. *Lucy in the Sky with Diamonds*. Sgt. Pepper's Lonely Hearts Club Band. Parlophone. 1967.
7. Becker, Ernest. *The Denial of Death*. Free Press. 1973.
8. Belfort, Jordan. *Way of the Wolf: Straight Line Selling: Master the Art of Persuasion, Influence, and Success*. Simon & Schuster. 2017.
9. Beyer, Adam. *Going Down.* Going Down. Drumcode. 2016.
10. Bible. *John 15:13*. n.d.
11. Brady, Tom. *The Greatest Comeback in Football History*. Howard Stern Interview. 2020.
12. Brown, Brene. *Daring Greatly.* Avery. 2015.
13. Brown, Brene. *The Anatomy of Trust*. Speech. 2019.
14. Buffett, Warren. *Warren Buffett's Success: What You Can Learn From it*. NDTV. 2015.
15. Castel, Marc. *Fiix Software.* n.d.
16. Castel, Mark. *AEI Speakers Bureau*. n.d.
17. Center for Addiction and Mental Health, The. *Crisis Resources*. n.d.
18. CheckPoint. *Global Mental Health Resources*. n.d.
19. Chesterton, G. K. *Heretics*. Dover Publications. 1905.
20. Chesterton, G. K. *The Everlasting Man.* Hodder & Stoughton. 1925.

21. **Clear, James.** *Atomic Habits: An Easy & Proven Way to Build Good Habits & Break Bad Ones.* **Avery. 2018.**
22. **Coelho, Paulo.** *The Alchemist.* **HarperTorch. 2006.**
23. **Deita, David.** *The Way Of The Superior Man: A Spiritual Guide to Mastering the Challenges of Women, Work, and Sexual Desire. 2004.*
24. **Dispenza, Joe.** *Breaking The Habit Of Being Yourself.* **Hay House Inc. 2013.**
25. **Dispenza, Joe.** *Morning Meditation.* **Morning And Evening Meditations. Fishpond. 2015.**
26. **Dispenza, Joe.** *Rewired.* **Gaia. 2019.**
27. **Einstein, Albert. Quotes. 1879-1955.**
28. **Ferriss, Tim.** *The 4-Hour Workweek.* **Crown Publishing Group. 2007.**
29. **Fiix Software.** *Careers.* **n.d.**
30. **Fly, Blake.** *Instagram: @ blakefly.* **n.d.**
31. **Gabriel, Iain.** *Instagram: @ iaingabriel.* **n.d.**
32. **Gandhi. Quotes. 1869-1948.**
33. **Godin, Seth.** *Linchpin: Are You Indispensable?.* **Portfolio. 2011.**
34. **Government of Canada.** *Mental health support: Get help.* **2021.**
35. **Gregoryk, Jerzy.** *Tim Ferris Show.* **Interview. 2017.**
36. **Haymen, Jesse Lee.** *Jack.org.* **n.d.**
37. **Hill, Napoleon.** *Think and Grow Rich.* **Napoleon Hill Foundation. 1937.**
38. **Hitchens, Christopher. Quotes. 1949-2011.**
39. **Jack.org.** *Bethere.org.* **n.d.**
40. **Jack.org.** *Jack Talks.* **n.d.**
41. **Jung, Carl. Quotes. 1875-1961.**
42. **Kent, Jack.** *There's No Such Thing as a Dragon.* **Random House Children's Books. 1975.**
43. **Kierkegaard, Soren. Quotes. 1813-1855.**
44. **Klangkarussell.** *Hey Maria Elderbrook Remix.* **Hey Maria Elderbrook Remix. Concord Music Publishing. 2016.**
45. **Kornfield, Jack.** *A Path with Heart: A Guide Through the Perils and Promises of Spiritual Life.* **Bantam. 1993.**
46. **Landmark Worldwide.** *Advanced Forum.* **n.d.**
47. **Landmark Worldwide.** *Self-Expression and Leader-*

ship Program. n.d.
48. Lebouf, Shia. *Just Do It.* Speech. 2015.
49. Marley, Bob. Quotes. 1945-1981.
50. Max, Tucker. *New York Times Best Seller, Tucker Max on Business, Fame, Women & Branding.* IKON-ICK Blank Canvas. Interview. 2020.
51. Nightingale, Earl. *The Strangest Secret*. Sound Wisdom. 1957.
52. Peterson, Jordan. *Slaying The Dragon Within Us.* Lecture. 2003.
53. Pollan, Michael. *Food Rules: An Eater's Manual.* Penguin Press. 2009.
54. Pollan, Michael. *How To Change Your Mind: What The New Science of Psychedelics Teaches Us About Consciousness, Dying, Addiction, Depression, and Transcendence*. Penguin Books. 2019.
55. Pressfield, Ethan. *The Warrior Ethos*. Black Irish Entertainment. 2011.
56. Richmond, Steve. *Men and Masculinity.* n.d.
57. Roberts, Gregory David. *Shantaram.* St. Martin's Griffin. 2005.
58. Rohn, Jim. *Learn This Skill Or Live A Mediocre Life.* YouTube. 1981.
59. Rohn, Jim. *The Seasons of Life*. Jim Rohn Intl. 1981.
60. Rohn, Jim. *The Ultimate Jim Rohn Collection*. Audible. n.d.
61. Rowden, Cole. Quotes. n.d.
62. Rumi. Quotes. 1207-1273.
63. Russ. *Money On Me*. Money On Me. 2021.
64. Scheinfeld, Robert. *Busting Loose From The Money Game*. Wiley. 2006.
65. Shafee, Armin. *Instagram: @ thearminshafee.* n.d.
66. Silverstein, Shel. *Everything On It.* HarperCollins. 2011.
67. Slater, AC. *Fly Kicks (Wax Motif Remix)*. This is Night Bass Vol 1. Night Bass Records. 2015.
68. Statistics Canada. *Suicide rates: An overview.* 2017.
69. Sterling, Justin. *Men's Weekend.* Sterling Institute. n.d.
70. Thoreau, Henry David. *Walden.* Ticknor and Fields. 1854.
71. Toastmasters International. *Find a Club*. n.d.

72. **Tolkien, J.R.R.** *The Fellowship of the Ring.* **George Allen & Unwin. 1954.**
73. **Tolkien, J.R.R.** *The Hobbit.* **George Allen & Unwin. 1937.**
74. **Tolle, Eckhart.** *The Power of Now: A Guide to Spiritual Enlightenment.* **New World Library. 1997.**
75. **Wachowski, Lana, et al.** *The Matrix.* **Warner Bros. Village. 1999.**
76. **Watts, Alan.** *Out of Your Mind*. **Alan Watts Audio Archives. n.d.**
77. **Wells, H.G.** *A Short History of the World*. **Cassell & Company. 1992.**
78. **Wertheimer, Max, et al.** *The Gestalt Principle.* **1923-1928.**
79. **Wikipedia.** *List of suicide crisis lines*. **2021.**
80. **Windeler, Eric.** *Instagram: @ ericwindeler*. **n.d.**
81. **World Health Organization.** *Suicide: one person dies every 40 seconds.* **2019.**
82. **WRLD, Juice.** *Bad Energy.* **Legends Never Die. Interscope. 2020.**
83. **WRLD, Juice.** *Legends Never Die.* **Interscope. 2020.**
84. **WRLD, Juice.** *On God*. **Death Race for Love. Interscope. 2019.**
85. **WRLD, Juice.** *Wishing Well.* **Legends Never Die. Interscope. 2020.**
86. **Zalucki, George.** *Profile of a Champion.* **George Zalucki. 1986.**
87. **Zalucki, George.** *The power of mindset*. **Speech. 2008.**
88. **Ziglar, Zig. Quotes. 1926-2012.**

About the Author

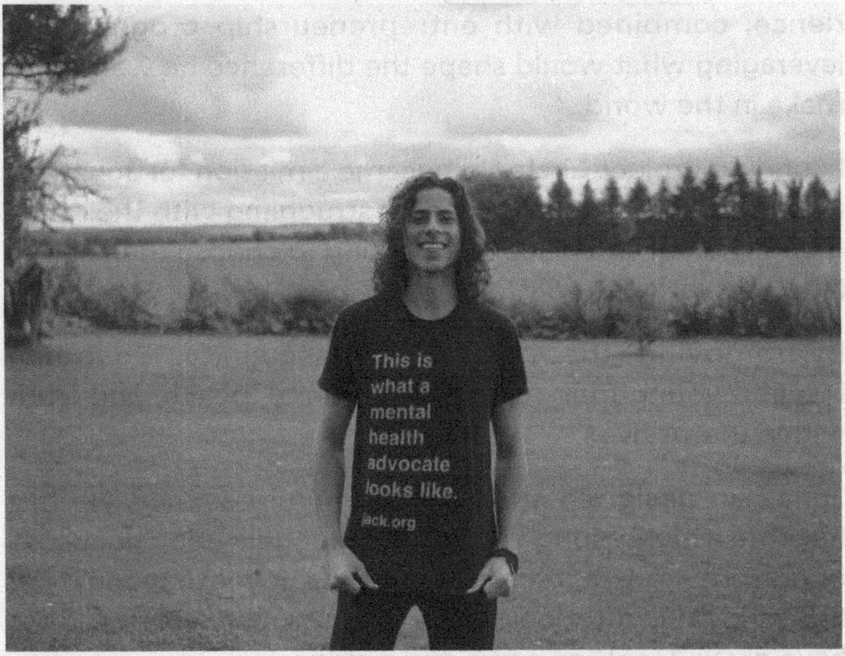

Jonathan Andrews speaks of "making peace with dragons." He's got a Knight's heart, but he's his own hero.

A passionate Youth Mental Health Champion and Award-Winning Speaker, Jonathan challenges young men to rip off their masks and reveal themselves to the men they trust in order to make them stronger. He wants to remove the shame and stigma of mental health struggle and reveal it for the growth opportunity it can be.

After being clinically diagnosed with depression and anxiety in high school, he knew that he himself had to shift and change to heal. He turned that healing into a mission... for all men, just like him, hiding in the shadows and afraid of their own dragons.

He dove into entrepreneurship programs and even became a Distinguished Toastmaster, Toastmasters International's highest honour, in 2018. With less than 1% of Toastmasters achieving this designation, Jonathan credits this experience, combined with entrepreneurship programs, in leveraging what would shape the difference he wanted to make in the world..

Founding Project Circle Up became a mission for Jonathan as he inspired hundreds of men, struggling with their own mental health and place in this world to choose themselves (and each other).

By removing the masks of masculinity, Jonathan inspired young men to find community, peace, and truth within themselves.

Jonathan designed a life of community service. He has become a highly sought-after Speaker delivering hundreds of presentations to tens of thousands of youth worldwide. Educational institutions and major corporate brands alike have given Jonathan a mic and a stage.

He continues to dedicate his time, energy, and resources to organizations inspiring and uplifting youth and men's mental health including the Special Olympics Ontario, Sterling Institute of Relationships, and Canada's leading charity for youth mental health education, Jack.org.

In 2020, Jonathan founded Project Circle Up, which includes a 10-week virtual wellness program with participants graduating across North and South America, Europe, and the Middle East.

His Podcast, Project Circle Up, aims at amplifying empowered masculinity by featuring the mental health journeys of men globally. His Podcast has achieved a global ranking as one of the top 10% most popular shows out of more than 2.5 million podcasts.

He currently resides wherever his journal and backpack take him... most likely a circle of men who are choosing the future of men's mental health; not to "man up," but to Circle Up.

Circle Up
By The Brotherhood

In many ways this entire book is simply an introduction. It's an introduction to me, to Circle Up, and to the broader challenges we as men face in respect to our mental health and masculinity. To be part of a men's team and learn more about how to implement the philosophy into your life, we embrace you:

Instagram: @projectcircleup **or** @jonathanfandrews
Email: jonathanandrewscircleup@gmail.com
Website: circleup.ca

LIFE TO PAPER
PUBLISHING INC.

Life to Paper Publishing Inc. (Life to Paper) is an independent publishing house, which helps diverse, mission-driven, heart-centred individuals put their life to paper and reach and inspire audiences and readers.

Life to Paper takes a unique approach to publishing, providing not only ghostwriting, editing and hybrid-publishing services, but also marketing, branding and public relations services, to help individuals take their story from "book I wrote once" to bestseller.

Thanks to our team and partners, we are able to distribute books worldwide that touch the lives and hearts of readers. We guide our authors to discover their unique gifts and empower them to start delivering these talents to the world; therefore, achieving their dream come true and beyond.

Life to Paper aims to allow others to see an author's deepest truths that guide them on a journey to stare directly into their own. We foster storytellers because we believe that "your story can be someone's spark", and change a life.

The Bookshop by Life to Paper is a physical bookstore, which serves the community of Buena Vista, Miami, Florida. We decided to open our doors even further, supporting local authors and artists and providing a place for future authors to commence working on their stories and workshop their pieces through our literary society. The Bookshop by Life to Paper is a place of inspiration and community, showcasing that, if you set your mind to it, you can write the book of your dreams, and we'll help you along the way.

Life to Legacy Foundation is Life to Paper Publishing's not-for-profit organization dedicated to educating and empowering individuals with courses, books and resources to write their life stories. We believe we can change the world one story at a time, and the Life to Legacy Foundation is our way of giving back to all the communities that deserve to have their stories shared.

CPSIA information can be obtained
at www.ICGtesting.com
Printed in the USA
LVHW032044191021
700895LV00008B/19/J

9 781777 373641